The Expert Guide to
Fertility

The Expert Guide to

Fertility

Boost
Your Chances for
Pregnancy

Joseph S. Sanfilippo, MD, MBA

with Aarti Kumar, MD

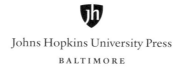

Johns Hopkins University Press

BALTIMORE

Disclaimer: The information provided is designed to assist in infertility evaluation and treatment. It is not to be taken as the way to evaluate the specific health problem you have. It is not designed to be a specific patient treatment plan. Your health care professional is the best person to provide you with evaluation and treatment for your specific problem. The stories are representative of actual patients, with names and details altered to protect their privacy.

© 2023 Johns Hopkins University Press
All rights reserved. Published 2023
Printed in the United States of America on acid-free paper
9 8 7 6 5 4 3 2 1

Johns Hopkins University Press
2715 North Charles Street
Baltimore, Maryland 21218
www.press.jhu.edu

All illustrations are by Jane Whitney. Figures 2.1, 2.2, 3.1, and 3.2 are based on illustrations by Natalie Nakles, MD. All photographs are courtesy of the authors.

Library of Congress Cataloging-in-Publication data is available.

ISBN 13: 978-1-4214-4705-6 (hc)
ISBN 13: 978-1-4214-4706-3 (pbk)
ISBN 13: 978-1-4214-4707-0 (ebook)

A catalog record for this book is available from the British Library.

Special discounts are available for bulk purchases of this book.
For more information, please contact Special Sales at specialsales@jh.edu.

Contents

Preface   vii

Preface

A Broadway musical, *The King and I*, has a song with the lyrics, "If you become a teacher, by your students you'll be taught." Let's modify that to, "When you become a doctor, by your patients you'll be taught."

We're Here for You

"I'm frustrated. Why me?" Many, many times we have heard this from patients. You are not alone on this daunting journey, which is often filled with detours. Fifteen percent of couples have a problem with infertility, which means 180 million people worldwide have fertility issues. But let's focus on you. We mean that sincerely. As teachers in medicine, we educate others to "be there" for their patients. And both of us have tried to be there for every one of our patients. This approach is the primary focus of this book: being there for you! What we have learned as health care professionals is to be there, in good times and in bad.

This book has been written to stand by your side on your journey toward fertility. The good news is that much progress has been made in assisting people who have difficulties getting pregnant. Years ago, we had only pills and injections to help women to ovulate. Now we can offer in vitro fertilization (IVF), and a couple with a decreased egg count, low sperm count, or maybe even no sperm (in their ejaculate) can achieve a pregnancy.

The surgical aspects have come a long way, too. We offer several procedures, including robotics, to put fallopian tubes back together following a tubal ligation, and it may be possible to surgically remove a fibroid or an overgrowth of endometrial tissue (endometriosis), conditions that may interfere with a woman's ability to become pregnant. If cancer has been diagnosed, we can freeze eggs, sperm, or ovarian or testicular tissue to allow a couple to have their own genetic child following cancer treatment.

Transgender patients can cryopreserve sperm or eggs for future fertility, thus allowing them to have their own genetic child. We can also freeze eggs for women who are not planning a pregnancy in the immediate future but want to retain that option, even to become pregnant at an age when their fertility might be reduced markedly.

One goal of this book is to equip you with a detailed understanding of your specific medical situation, what tests may be needed, and the treatment options and resources available. The book is also meant to improve communication between you and your health care provider. We provide you with resources that you can check out to learn more about infertility. Illustrations are included to aid you in understanding infertility evaluation and treatment.

We address areas such as how to prepare for conception, emphasizing lifestyle, healthy living, and ideal BMI (body mass index), as well as practices to avoid, such as smoking, vaping, and using marijuana. We provide hope for men, including the option to seek expertise from a trained expert in male infertility and urology. We provide details related to female infertility, such as what tests and treatment options are available. Having uterine fibroids may prevent a woman from becoming pregnant or complicate a pregnancy, and we explain the treatment options. For pelvic pain and endometriosis, we explore when surgery is needed and what medical treatment options exist. Polycystic ovary syndrome (PCOS) affects 10% of women, making it the most common endocrine problem in females. We provide an understanding of the problem and the treatment options.

Overall, the book is designed to provide you with a better understanding of what it might take to become pregnant. We arm you with the information you need to be more involved in your care and the decision-making process. We encourage you to see the light at the end of the tunnel. Best wishes to you for every success!

The Expert Guide to
Fertility

Chapter 1

Christie's Story

A Personal Infertility Experience

"It only takes once," said my mama when preparing me for what could happen with premarital intercourse. A pregnancy, in her mind, required only one chance encounter before a positive test. Fast-forward 20 years. I am no longer 16 years old and no longer believe it only takes once. I know much better now. At 36, I know that it takes 11 rounds of intra-uterine insemination (IUI), 5 rounds of in vitro fertilization (IVF), 91 retrieved follicles (precursors to developing eggs), 4 failed transfers, 4 different fertility clinics in 4 different states, more than $250,000, a husband who loves me unconditionally, and me . . . someone who isn't giving up on the dream of becoming a mother, however that happens.

Preventing pregnancy was always a part of my plan until I was married. I started my "serious" dating career after college. The effect of birth control pills on my hormones made me so crazy that I was only on them for a total of five months my entire adult life. I didn't like introducing chemicals into my body. Being extremely in tune with my body made "natural family planning"—or basically just knowing by my cervical fluids when I should be extra careful—an easy way to avoid pregnancy.

When I met my husband, I always thought a honeymoon baby would be fun—and if I'm being honest, I thought it would be impressive. I was so certain that my lack of birth control, my on-time period each month, and my attention to my body would/should result in getting pregnant easily. The first month that it didn't work I wasn't worried, as we were still within the honeymoon phase. The second month, I started to do handstands after intercourse and then lie still for at least 20 minutes with my hips on a pillow. The third month, I let my husband know we had entered the "trying" phase. The fourth month is when I began experiencing feelings of confusion, disappointment, self-questioning, and eagerness for results. As a woman, wasn't this something that was supposed to be easy? Wasn't this the one thing I could do that my husband couldn't? I went to my OB (obstetrician-gynecologist) and lied. I told her we had been trying for 7+ months so she would direct me to the next steps. I didn't have the time—or rather, like most type-A women, I didn't want to use my time waiting for some textbook standard of trying for 12 months before clinical assistance. I was a unique case that needed a faster timeline. It never dawned on me the actual amount of time I would end up waiting.

My original OB-GYN spent only a few minutes chatting with me about my body and my plan. "Have you tried Clomid? Have you gone to a fertility clinic? They are factories, you're young [I was 31 at the time]; you'll be pregnant in no time." So many things were wrong about this. (1) I didn't like the quick turn to drugs. Remember that part about not being on birth control pills? (2) She didn't ask about my history: Had I ever been pregnant? How were my periods? When were we having intercourse? Was I ovulating? (3) There was no suggestion of testing to learn more.

At this early stage, I was still thinking that a quick fix was obtainable. I didn't have fertility problems; my husband's swimmers just hadn't met my lady eggs at the right time yet. I knew this wasn't going to take long—I was so healthy and young. Trying to get pregnant at 31 is not an outlandish idea. I started calculating my due dates each month.

The recommended clinic was worse than the OB-GYN had been. There was no real investigation of my past. I found myself waiting for someone to hear me explain how painful my periods had been since my first cycle and immediately understand why it wasn't working. They didn't. My husband and I took days off work, boarded our dogs, spent the night in hotels, and naively walked into the clinic for four IUI cycles, each time with the same hope. With no positive results, they said the next steps were an invasive laparoscopy (a surgical procedure where a camera was inserted into my belly). I put my foot down. I'm not your run-of-the-mill patient, and I am certainly not a one-size-fits-all type of gal. If you can't ask me about my period, I can't be your patient. We walked out the door and found another clinic. Locally this time. Whew.

This new local clinic came through a reference from a friend who knew the doctor, who was a real gem. During our initial consultation—scheduled for 45 minutes—she didn't look at her watch once during the hour and 15 minutes that we peppered her with questions. We asked lots of questions. Why is this not working? How can you tell what we should do? What options do we have? How much does it cost? How long will this take? Probably 5 to 7 IUIs (you really do start to lose count) and 1 laparoscopy later, with our new doctor, it was time for IVF. After 2 rounds of IVF, 27 retrieved follicles, 2 named embryos (don't name your embryos!), 3 cleared genetic screenings, 3 failed transfers, and being 2 years older, we moved on to another clinic.

This time, we packed our suitcases, boarded a plane (a few times), and headed to the team of doctors in another state who were supposed to be pretty smart. By now we were starting to understand the business of IVF. Costs were higher, but so was the quality of care. I had my own finance liaison (you need that when you're paying that much!), my own nurse, and my own doctor, who had limited patients. I received daily calls with lab updates, appointments ran on time, and the retrievals were like clockwork. We lived in a hotel for eight days each time. During our first retrieval, they retrieved 12 eggs. At this point I didn't know how many were mature and how many were pre- or post-mature. All I know is that only *one* follicle fertilized, which meant we only had one shot of this egg going through the genetic/chromosomal screening that we had planned.

If there was ever a time to believe my mama about something only taking once, this was it. That mighty little follicle turned into a blast, an embryo, and made it through the testing. We had one. We only needed one. This was it. Until it wasn't.

Even though we were distraught and exhausted (we didn't realize then what true exhaustion was), we were impressed enough by the clinic that we were willing to try again. This time they said their entire team of 50+ doctors were going to review my case at their weekly meeting and decide on the next best plan for me, one that we were hoping would be the sure bet. We did the bag-packing, plane-boarding, and hotel-living thing again. This time, the retrieval produced eight eggs. Not enough for a football team, but I could put five on a basketball court. When they went to inseminate this group, *zero* were mature. Not one of the embryos were mature enough—in spite of them measuring 20 millimeters—to inseminate. All of that effort, time, money, and 50 doctors deciding on a plan, and that's the card we were dealt. The hardest part of that was calling my parents. If you haven't realized, parents get pretty involved in your hopes, too.

What on earth had happened? The flood of "whys?" took over. We were told that the fastest and most economical way to become parents was to find an egg donor. Let me pause here and pay tribute to all the people like me, who never in their wildest dreams imagined being in this situation. No one ever thinks they will be told that donor eggs are the only answer. No one thinks that they will find themselves in the IVF waiting room. No one thinks that they will need professional help doing what humans have done for years, successfully procreating without having to split the atom—or rather, the egg.

Time for a real time-out. We were shocked. We took our Marriott points and went home. Dumbfounded, speechless, lost, with no idea how to find our way out of this ring of purgatory.

So, we took a few months off from trying to get pregnant with no outside medical help. There have been few times during our marriage that we have made love without me thinking about if this time was going to result in a baby. We went the holistic approach. Acupuncture two to four times per month. Fertility massages (yes, those are a thing), vitamins, diet changes, meditation, and more. The vitamin and diet changes were minimal, as I have been on and off of dairy, gluten, sugar, and caffeine for most of my life. Vitamins have been a staple for me since I was a kid. This wasn't new; I just wasn't sure what to do other than get my body in tip-top shape. After a while, I realized, it likely wasn't only my body that needed attention, my mind could use a restart, too. I started doing morning meditations. I wasn't leading retreats, but 10 minutes at the start of the day was enough to get my mind right. I increased my communication with the universe and with the little babies out there, one of which would become mine. I assured them how much we already loved them—that Mama and Daddy were not perfect, but we were going to love and care for them the best we know how.

With my body becoming a temple, my mind staying focused and positive, I finally followed the advice of two friends and my previous fertility doctor and headed west to a renowned clinic with impressive stats and a no-nonsense approach. We went for a full-day workup where every fertility test in the book was performed. At the end of the probing day—for both me and my husband—we met the doctor to review the results. Everything looked great. I rolled my eyes because, honestly, everything had always looked great. My fallopian tubes were open. My egg reserve was good for my age. My uterine lining looked great. What did cause them to pause, though, was the number of follicles they saw on initial testing. They saw about six, give or take. One side had four, the other had around two or so. We were back to it only taking only one to fulfill our dream.

In that meeting, the doctor ran through the numbers and statistics—finally, a fertility language my husband could understand. When the numbers were run, the statistics calculated, our chances of getting one healthy, chromosomally normal embryo were *small*. So small that we walked out the front door and both agreed that we would likely not be back to this place.

What they also told us in that meeting was that we had the option to do two to three retrievals in a row. Get some good blasts (day 5 embryos, which consist of 100–200 cells) the first time (maybe one or two), do the retrieval protocol again, get another one to two blasts, do it again, and try to get a total of four to six embryos to test genetically. While this approach seemed logical, it also seemed like it would take forever and be expensive. It felt like these people were throwing months around like I was in my twenties and dollars around like our funds were unlimited.

As if on cue, we got home and regrouped. What did I feel in my gut? What was I willing to subject myself to? What were our options? This decision took months—again!

Fast forward, we did more research, and I found a minimal stimulation approach I wanted to try. Less drugs, less toxins in my body as we tried to grow my eggs. When I called around to a few clinics, I wasn't getting a good feeling. So I called out west again and asked if they offered this protocol. They said this is what the doctor had mentioned months ago. Sometimes you don't hear what is happening around you when you are in your dark place from receiving bad news.

We were ready. I felt in my heart of hearts that I was a healthy woman capable of creating and carrying a child. Before we entertained any more ideas about adoption, egg donors, surrogates, or being the "fun" aunt and uncle with two incomes and no kids, we decided to give it one last shot. This was it. This was for all the marbles. This was the last hurrah, the final approach.

This clinic, finally, put an emphasis on pre-procedure vitamins for both me and my husband. Nothing was going to be quick about this process, but I was grateful that they wanted my body and my cells to be in prime condition before giving them our last IVF-allotted dollars. At last, it was time to start the priming for the retrieval. Belly injections, little blue tabs of estradiol, lab work, and baseline ultrasounds. We were back in the game. The stakes were high, but we were practically pros at retrievals at this point.

My ultrasounds were showing good numbers—promising follicles—and good sizes. But let's take the word "promising" out. I don't think they ever used it. If they would have, it probably would have sent me through the roof because that's one of those words that gives unfounded hope, and while we need hope in this process, we don't need false hope. There are no promises in this line of experiences. Follicles aren't promising until you deliver.

Because there were good-looking follicles on both sides, more than what they anticipated, we took the trigger shot. It is a weird process because for the next 24–36 hours you just sit and wait and pretend to be normal while you are waiting to see if your luck is about to change for the better. Retrieval morning came, and they got every single one of the 26 follicles out. Groggy but happy in the recovery room, I started to think we had a chance.

Status call after status call, the odds were in our favor. Four of the follicles had taken to the insemination. An update a week later: three of them had made it to day 6. Yes, people outside of the IVF world probably think that going from 26 to 3 isn't really a good thing, but all of us in the club know that those are numbers to happily take any day. Next up was genetic testing. Somehow, they made it. All three tested chromosomally normal. We had three viable embryos. This was good. Very good.

Round two came. At this point, while I was thrilled with our previous results, I was less than thrilled to be going through this *again*. Did I really need to be starting the retrieval process for a sixth time? Weren't three embryos enough? Couldn't we have more kids than we had beds available with what we have from round one? They said that, on average, you need two healthy embryos for every one healthy pregnancy. If we wanted two children, we needed at least one more. At this point, what was another two months? What was another couple of thousands of dollars? I thought it was a lot to ask, actually. I was tired of spending money on medications, and I was tired of my life revolving around injection schedules and apologizing for being erratic because of the hormones. But it was the youngest I was ever going to be. Our logic was this: If we transferred one embryo now and it didn't take, we would need to use another one. If the second one took, I would be pregnant and deliver, and then if we wanted another baby after that, we would have only one embryo left. So . . . I would be two years older and possibly needing to start from scratch again. Being a professional IVFer is not part of my career plan. We decided to do round 2 in quick succession.

The second retrieval showed good quality and quantity. Not as many as the first time, but I was checking out mentally and not very engaged in this one, so I wasn't too concerned. I ended up triggering early—it looked like the follicles were being overachievers even when Mommy felt like skipping school. The retrieval resulted in 14 retrieved follicles. Already our numbers were down. This was precisely our pattern over the past six years—high retrieval number, few quality eggs. We knew these numbers weren't great for us. We felt a little deflated, but honestly, I was just ready to stop living in a hotel room and for my pants to fit again. We called home and gave the report that this trip wasn't as successful as the previous one, but either way, we gave it our best.

The lab called us and said that seven follicles were inseminated. They were going to let them grow, and they would call us back in a week. A week later, we got the miraculous news that four had made it, and two weeks later, those four had also been deemed as chromosomally normal.

What? How? We officially had seven healthy and normal embryos waiting to become babies. I cried and cried and cried. I felt confident that I was finally going to be a mama someday. Everything in my world turned on its head. This time for the better.

My outlook on life changed. People could tell me they were pregnant, and I could be around babies and people who wouldn't stop talking about their kids (please nudge me hard if this is ever me). I wasn't pregnant yet, but I sure did feel like I would be one day soon. Seven? Lucky number seven? Sure, whatever—it would have been "lucky four" if we had only four.

The Kentucky Derby was running a few weeks before our transfer. My husband, the numbers and statistics guy, loves to bet the ponies. I prefer to dress up, people watch, and keep my money in my purse—or pay for IVF. This particular Derby, I was charged with making the group bet. The bet was $80 on one horse. More than I had ever put on one horse in my life. To my surprise, the horse won. The group made me place the bet on the next race too. And that horse also won. I knew that day that our double-income, child-free, and two–"fur baby" family was about to change. Luck was with us. Science seemed to be with us. The universe was with us. Evidently, it was time.

With my transfer priming protocol complete, it was time to choose our embryo. Loving them all equally (already sounding like a parent), we made our choice, crossed our fingers, and watched the little guy (the size of a period on a page, maybe smaller) appear on the big screen. There he was. Could this be it?

Cautiously optimistic, we waited. And waited. Hell hath no fury like an IVF woman waiting for results. We were on edge, giddy, nervous, and realizing nothing else mattered other than what the lab sent in the results. I used a new lab for my HCG (human chorionic gonadotropin) test. A lab that emails you the results the same time they send the physician results. I saw the email. I called my husband off the golf course and asked if he wanted me to open the results and read them for us or wait until the doctor called. Not an ice cube's chance in hell were we waiting one more minute. I looked, he looked, the ranges looked . . . good? To be pregnant, they want you to have an HCG level of 50 or above. Mine was 295. For the first time in my life, I was pregnant.

As of today, I am 10 weeks and 6 days pregnant. I say my prayers every morning, thanking the universe that the babe is still with us and asking if he can stay. It's still, as you realize, out of my hands.

It almost annoys me to end on this note with you. When asked why I never joined support groups of other women going through IVF during the past six years, my response was always honest. It would be too hard and frustrating when one of them would get pregnant. I always found more comfort with people in the trenches with me, not when someone crawled out and left me behind. So, I won't end here to tell you that all stories, even those that cost too much money and take too long, have a happy ending. Yours may or may not. I hope more than anything that you find happiness in however your story ends—or begins.

I'll say that my marriage is stronger, and I have a deeper appreciation for how strong I am. I know you are strong, too. Stronger than you imagine. This process isn't for the faint of heart or for those who are unsure of what they want. Fertility journeys take all of you, and then they ask for more. And because of your grit, your determination, your willingness to do whatever it takes for your baby that isn't here yet, you give it everything you have and then some. Your course might change, your perspective might change, and you will certainly change, but what you want doesn't change. My heart and support go out to every person reading this and wondering how their story will begin and end.

I am hopeful that you find answers, comfort, and resources in this book. It is chock-full of clinical information, suggestions, advice from a respected fertility doctor, and real-life accounts of fertility experiences. This doctor is often my first call when I want the truth, when I want answers, and when I want to know what he would suggest to his own daughter. This book was written by a team of brilliant and kind doctors— exactly who you want in your corner as you're figuring out the most mystifying chapter of your life.

Tomorrow morning, when I give myself my last progesterone injection with a two-inch needle into my bruised bottom, it will be for all of you, all of us. It will be for every woman who has wanted a family but couldn't or didn't. For those who came before us who didn't have the medical options we have now. For all of us who have wanted this but have to take the long way there. The long way isn't always the worst way— sometimes it's the only and most rewarding way.

Thank you for reading my story. I hope you've been inspired not to give up.

With love and endless admiration for you,
Christie Leigh

Postscript: Miracle IVF baby W was born in February 2022.

Chapter 2

Enhancing Your Chances

Optimizing Natural Fertility

IT HAS BEEN A TRYING DAY at work with my 5-year-old kindergarteners but oddly satisfying, too, since I can't imagine doing anything else. Lately I've been thinking about starting a family of my own. Steve, my partner, has always said he's committed whenever I'm ready. I know I want to expand my family, but I want to make sure I know what to do to maximize my chances of having a healthy pregnancy.—*Carmen*

What You Need to Know about Preconception Counseling

Why Is It Important?

The goal of **preconception counseling** is to maximize the chances of getting pregnant by understanding the process of ovulation, conception, and the factors that influence a healthy pregnancy outcome. Proceeding with preconception screening and taking steps to enhance your fertility is ideal. Talking to your health care provider regarding pregnancy planning and timing as well as being evaluated for items that could interfere with your pregnancy is time well spent. It is important to develop a relationship with both your OB-GYN and primary care

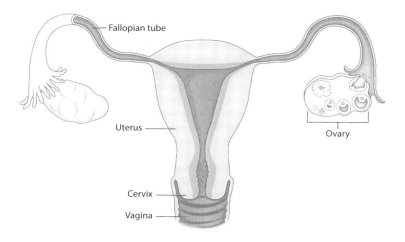

FIGURE 2.1.
Anatomy of the female reproductive system.

provider, as this journey is challenging. The members of your health care team are important partners. Get comfortable with them, and consider following their recommendations.

What Do I Need to Know about Ovulation?

To enhance your chances of conception, it is important to understand how your natural ovulation cycle works (see figure 2.1 for the basic anatomy of the female reproductive system). **Ovulation** is when the body releases a mature egg into the fallopian tubes, giving the sperm that have traveled into the fallopian tubes the opportunity to fertilize the egg. Generally, the time of ovulation is 14 days prior to the onset of your period. Therefore timing is everything.

The first signs of ovulation may be mid-cycle watery vaginal discharge. The watery aspect of the discharge serves as a ladder for the sperm to enter the uterus and ultimately get to the fallopian tubes. Sperm can survive 5–10 days in the reproductive tract. It is hard to identify one optimal day for intercourse, but starting from the first signs of ovulation, couples may want to have intercourse three days in a row or every other day for three days around ovulation. Some couples prefer to have sex daily over the ovulatory window.

How Do I Know When I'm Ovulating?

There are a number of methods to track a **fertile period**. The simplest is basal body temperature (BBT) monitoring, which means taking your temperature daily and noting a low point or dip right before ovulation. Once ovulation occurs, BBT rises because progesterone, the key hormone produced following ovulation, slightly increases a woman's body temperature. Ovulation predictor kits can help pinpoint when you are ovulating. Another device is Mira, which provides home fertility monitoring of estrogen and LH (luteinizing hormone), which peak around ovulation. There are also multiple fertility smartphone apps that can be used to identify ovulation, serving as an aid for timing of intercourse either for pregnancy or as a mode of contraception.

Below are some of the fertility apps that you can use to monitor ovulation:

- Clue Period & Cycle Tracker
- Flo Period & Ovulation Tracker
- Glow
- Fertility Friend
- Natural Cycles
- Ovia Fertility & Cycle Tracker
- Period Tracker by GP Apps

How Does My Health Affect a Potential Pregnancy?

Good maternal health can improve pregnancy results. Being in your healthiest condition as it relates to lifestyle is beneficial for your well-being and can affect both your chances of getting pregnant and the health of the pregnancy. Visiting your primary care provider, including your obstetrician-gynecologist (OB-GYN), prior to getting pregnant is

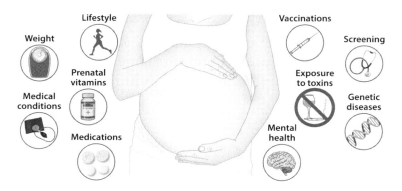

FIGURE 2.2.
Factors that influence fertility.

helpful because multiple preventative measures can be addressed for a healthy pregnancy. The best time for a preconception appointment is three to six months before trying to get pregnant.

Topics to Discuss with Your Doctor

Your doctor will obtain your full medical history, as there are many factors that can affect your ability to get pregnant (figure 2.2). Below are some of the things your health care provider will discuss with you during preconception counseling.

Lifestyle (Diet and Exercise)

Your doctor may ask you questions about your diet and exercise habits. For a healthy diet, we recommend that you follow the government guidelines listed in the Resources section (page 197). In addition to eating right, you should exercise regularly. The weekly exercise goal for a healthy woman should be 150 minutes of moderate physical activity.

Weight

Body mass index (BMI) is a value used to describe weight (see categories below). Being underweight can be associated with low-birth-weight babies and preterm birth. Obesity can lead to a higher-risk pregnancy and can affect fetal intrauterine growth. BMI is calculated based upon a person's height and weight, and can be estimated using the following online calculator: https://www.cdc.gov/healthyweight/assessing/bmi/adult _bmi/english_bmi_calculator/bmi_calculator.html.

- Normal weight BMI: 18.5 to 24.9
- Underweight BMI: less than 18.5
- Overweight BMI: 25 to 29.9
- Obese BMI: 30 or greater

A BMI of 30 or greater is associated with a number of problems during pregnancy. These complications include gestational diabetes, growth restriction of fetus, preeclampsia, the fetus's shoulder getting stuck at delivery (shoulder dystocia), and miscarriage. Ideally, a woman with a BMI of 30 or higher will reduce her weight before getting pregnant.

Vitamins and Nutrients

The first trimester of pregnancy (the first 13 weeks) is critical to organ development, so all pregnant women are strongly recommended to take a supplemental prenatal vitamin that includes folic acid. Folic acid is important because it can help prevent brain and spinal birth defects of the baby. Other crucial nutrients for a healthy pregnancy include calcium, iron, and vitamins A, B_{12}, B complex, and D. Your health care provider may recommend that you take additional vitamins or nutrients.

Herbals

You might be wondering whether herbal preparations could benefit your pregnancy. In the absence of reliable scientific studies, it may be best to avoid these supplements unless your doctor recommends them. Herbal preparations could interfere with other medications your health care providers prescribe.

Medical Conditions

Chronic conditions such as asthma, diabetes, high blood pressure, thyroid disease, seizures, and blood clotting disorders require monitoring and control prior to conception. During your pregnancy, your health care provider will closely monitor and treat these conditions as well.

For women with diabetes, we use hemoglobin A1c (Hgb A1c) as a good marker of overall glucose metabolism. Glucose metabolism is the conversion of sugar into energy, which is essential to healthy cell growth and function. Having an Hgb A1c level of below 5.7% is ideal for both mom and baby.

Immunologic conditions such as rheumatoid arthritis or lupus will require you to work closely with your health care provider. You may need to see a maternal fetal medicine specialist even before you get pregnant.

If you have high blood pressure (BP), discuss with your doctor what medications you are taking, as some BP medications are not advised during pregnancy, including beta blockers (atenolol) and ACE inhibitors (captopril or lisinopril). Many times, labetalol, nifedipine, or methyldopa are prescribed for pregnant women with high BP, but this is a decision your doctor will make with you.

Thyroid disorders (hypothyroidism and hyperthyroidism) that are not well controlled can be related to infertility and can cause miscarriage. Work with your doctor to decide the best thyroid-stimulating hormone (TSH) level for you. A TSH level of 2.5 or less is often ideal.

Medications

Review all the medications you currently take with your health care provider, and tell them you are planning to get pregnant. Each medication has pregnancy guidelines or at least correlative research study data that address safety during pregnancy.

Vaccinations

A health care provider will review your immunizations and determine whether you should receive any necessary vaccinations. In particular, immunity to German measles (rubella) and ideally chickenpox (varicella) is important prior to getting pregnant, as these viruses can be transmitted to the fetus and lead to detrimental outcomes. In case you have to be vaccinated or require a booster shot for German measles (known as MMR, for measles, mumps, and rubella vaccination) or chicken pox (varicella vaccination), then you should not plan pregnancy for one month after each injection, as these are live vaccines and can have a detrimental effect on the fetus. The following are recommended vaccinations prior to pregnancy:

- Chicken pox (varicella)
- Flu (influenza)
- German measles (rubella)
- Hepatitis B
- Measles
- Mumps
- Tdap (tetanus toxoid, diphtheria, pertussis)

Screening

Your health care provider may order additional screening before you become pregnant. In addition to an annual gynecological exam, you may have tests for sexually transmitted infections, including HIV, if indicated.

Your doctor may ask you questions about your home life. Intimate partner violence is a concern, as is reproductive coercion. If you are experiencing violence in your relationship or feel pressured to become pregnant, let your doctor know.

Exposure to Toxins

Toxins like tobacco, alcohol, marijuana, and illegal drugs can cause birth defects, inadequate fetal development, preterm delivery, and still-born birth. Alcohol is especially harmful. According to the American College of Obstetricians and Gynecologists, "There is no safe amount of alcohol to drink when pregnant." Toxin exposure includes secondary smoke, meaning your partner and other people around you can also create a poor environment for the baby. Environmental toxins like lead and mercury (which are found in the tissues of some fish—swordfish, shark, king mackerel, and tilefish) are also harmful to fetal development and should be avoided during pregnancy.

Genetic Diseases

Your genetic history and that of your partner or family is important because you may be a carrier for a genetic problem that can be passed on to the baby. If you undergo in vitro fertilization (IVF), preimplantation genetic testing may be indicated to test the embryo for genetic disorders. (For more on preimplantation genetic testing, see chapter 14.)

Mental Health

It is important to monitor your mental health, as pregnancy can be very taxing, both physically and mentally. If you have anxiety, depression, or another psychological or psychiatric diagnosis, it is important to work with your health care team and your support system as you embark on this pregnancy journey. Depression and anxiety are best controlled before getting pregnant, as is addressing any necessary medications. By having a discussion about your mental health with your providers, they can perform screening for depression and anxiety before you get pregnant.

Jolena's Story

ONE LOOK AT MY DESK at work will tell you I am a well-organized person. I like my coffee at around 9 a.m. and always leave home after a good, nutritious breakfast. My male partner makes fun of me and says I'm "too obsessed with working out," but I actually look forward to my spin classes. Recently, we have been thinking seriously about trying to get pregnant. True to my organized approach to life, we have decided to see a doctor for preconception counseling. I contacted my gynecologist, whose office staff suggested I see the physician assistant (PA) to get in sooner. The PA was great and told me it was a good idea to plan ahead. At my appointment, I told her we are thinking of getting pregnant in the next year. She asked my age and explained that age is important because it can affect how long you try to get pregnant before seeking medical help. What I remember is, if someone is under 35, it may take a year to conceive, and for someone over 35, if conception doesn't happen after six months, then an infertility evaluation is in order.

She conducted a detailed medical history and advised if I had any chronic illnesses like diabetes, high blood pressure, or thyroid problems, then they needed to be well controlled before I try. Thank heavens I am in good health! She checked in with me about partner violence. Fortunately, he is the love of my life and treats me like a queen. We talked about nutrition, exercise, and about ideally having a BMI of less than 25. She emphasized that I should take prenatal vitamins to increase my folic acid levels for two to three months before attempting to get pregnant. She then told me about screening for cystic fibrosis, SMA (spinal muscular atrophy), and Fragile X syndrome, especially if there is any related family history. We talked about whether I took birth control pills, about family genetic problems, and if I'd ever had a blood clot in my legs or chest, as such history could mean predisposition to blood clots during pregnancy.

Next, she brought up vaccinations and how they should be up to date. She handed me a list that included rubella (German measles), DPT (diphtheria, pertussis, and tetanus), and influenza and suggested I get a COVID-19 vaccination, too. Then we talked about

Zika and avoiding those places where it was prevalent. We discussed the harmful impact of smoking and marijuana for the fetus and pregnancy in general. She cautioned against eating too much fish and the dangers of exposure to mercury.

I mentioned to her about my cycle, which is 28–30 days, "like clockwork." She said that my ovulation should be 14 days before my period and we should time sex accordingly. She reminded me to keep track of my periods, as that would be important in dating the pregnancy.

I felt overwhelmed after the visit but was glad that it was so thorough! It was worth the time and effort to meet our PA. We are going to do what she suggested and are excited to follow up on her suggestions.

• TAKEAWAY POINTS •

Plan ahead (three to six months) of when you want to start trying to become pregnant.

Begin taking prenatal vitamins several months before pregnancy.

Focus on maintaining a healthy lifestyle (diet and exercise).

Ask your health care provider to recommend screening tests.

Avoid smoking, vaping, alcohol, marijuana, and illegal drugs.

Plan early visits to your doctor or other provider to monitor pregnancy.

• KEY WORDS •

body mass index (BMI)
fertile period
ovulation
preconception counseling

Chapter 3

Against All Odds

Female Infertility

MY LIFE HAS BEEN PRETTY GOOD so far. I am the leading supervisor at a software company, married to my best friend Ravi, and have a pet cat, Butterscotch. Ravi and I decided a while ago that we were finally ready to have kids. It has been a frustrating six months of using multiple ovulation predictor kits to find the "perfect" time, and yet I continue to get my stupid period. I know I am 38, but I really thought I could still get pregnant. I have always practiced safe sex, I work out regularly, eat healthy, and haven't had a drink since we started this process. What am I doing wrong? Even my older sister got pregnant at 38 the first time she tried!

Ravi continues to comfort me and says he loves me no matter what, but I know that it's important to us that we figure out what is wrong. We have recently found a reproductive endocrinologist—an infertility expert—who is our only hope.
—*Mahir*

What You Need to Know about Getting Pregnant

Several parts of your reproductive anatomy need to work together for you to become pregnant. The timing and accurate confirmation of pregnancy are also important.

Reproductive Anatomy

A woman's reproductive system is composed of ovaries, fallopian tubes, and a uterus. Each organ works in concert to initiate the menstrual cycle and possibly produce a pregnancy.

Ovaries. Each month, one of your ovaries releases an egg. If the egg is not fertilized, you get your period.

Fallopian tubes. The fallopian tubes transport the eggs from the ovaries to the uterus. Fertilization occurs in the tube where the egg meets the sperm.

Uterus. The fertilized egg rolls in a manner that has been described as moving like a bowling ball into the uterus and implants on the uterine lining.

Timing Sex with Ovulation

Ovulation predictor kits are helpful to pinpoint the best time for sex when you want to become pregnant. The American Society for Reproductive Medicine has additional recommendations for maximizing your chances of getting pregnant, including the timing of when you have sex and how your vaginal discharge can indicate that you are ovulating.

Having sex three days in a row or every other day, beginning with the first sign of ovulation until ovulation is over, is recommended because sperm can live in the female reproductive tract for six to seven days, depending on a variety of factors. One sign ovulation is beginning is having a vaginal discharge with a watery, egg-white consistency.

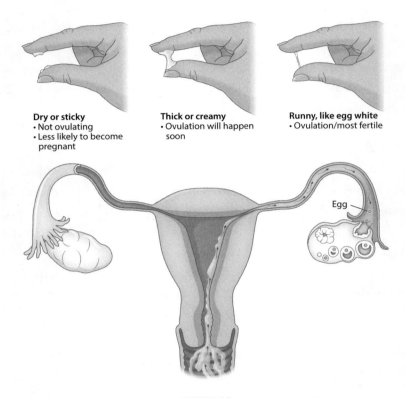

Dry or sticky
• Not ovulating
• Less likely to become pregnant

Thick or creamy
• Ovulation will happen soon

Runny, like egg white
• Ovulation/most fertile

Egg

FIGURE 3.1.
Cervical mucus at different stages of the menstrual cycle, and sperm migration through the reproductive tract.

Many women have an increase in cervical mucus and thus increased vaginal discharge when they are ovulating (figure 3.1).

Once your period is late, obtain a pregnancy test and follow up with your health care provider.

The Process of Getting Pregnant

Every month, the above components come together when the ovary develops one or more eggs in preparation for ovulation. When you reach mid-cycle, the increase in cervical mucus optimizes the chances of sperm entering the uterus. The mucus acts like a ladder for the sperm to travel from the vagina into the uterus. From the uterus, the sperm travels to the end of the fallopian tube, where it meets the egg for fertilization. Although sperm can live up to 6 to 7 days in a woman's body and result in a pregnancy, there is a limited window for fertilization of the egg to take place. Finally, the fertilized egg travels into the uterus and, 6 to 10 days later, the now tiny embryo implants in the lining of the uterus.

What Is Female Infertility?

Infertility affects an estimated 10% of women globally. This translates to 6 million women aged 15 to 44 in the United States and 48 million worldwide, according to the Centers for Disease Control and Prevention (CDC). Although peak fertility takes place when women are in their early to mid-20s, many women are postponing pregnancy to a later age. When you are ready to become pregnant, it is wise to seek **preconception counseling** sooner rather than later. Ask your primary care physician or OB-GYN for recommendations about preconception counseling. You can also check with your health insurance carrier for suggestions about counseling.

In medicine we use the term "advanced maternal age" for a woman 35 or older who is trying to achieve pregnancy. A woman's egg supply starts to diminish beginning at age 35 and slowly decreases thereafter. Therefore the woman's age is one metric for determining whether a successful pregnancy will occur. Issues regarding male infertility are covered in chapter 4.

Infertility is defined slightly differently depending on the woman's age. If you are under the age of 35 and have been unable to conceive after trying for one year, or if you are 35 or older and have been unable to conceive after trying for six months, you are considered to be experiencing infertility.

What Causes Female Infertility?

There are multiple causes of infertility, many of which have been studied and can be addressed. Sometimes the cause is unknown, or what is termed "unexplained infertility."

Anatomic Causes

Cervix. The cervix is an important part of the reproductive system and can be involved in several different types of infertility. Sperm enter the uterus through the cervix after being deposited in the vagina. If a woman can menstruate, then sperm can get through the cervix and journey on up to the fallopian tube, where fertilization occurs. Surgical treatment for an abnormal pap smear (such as a loop electrosurgical excision procedure, or LEEP) may cause scarring of the cervix, which could interfere with fertilization. It is helpful to rule out the possibility that a LEEP causes scarring; you should discuss this with your doctor.

Ovaries. A woman is born with all the eggs she will ever have in her ovaries. The eggs lie dormant and at early stages of development until after puberty. When a woman ovulates, an egg is released and flows into the fallopian tube, where fertilization occurs. The fertilized egg then travels into the uterus and implants on the uterine wall. Some women have a decreased egg supply, or ovarian reserve. This condition is common starting at age 35 but may occur prematurely. Some experience anovulation, which is the absence of ovulation. Difficulty with ovulation can be caused by:

- Hormonal disturbances such as thyroid abnormalities or poorly controlled diabetes
- Improper signals from the brain's pituitary gland to the ovaries

Remember: It's important to time intercourse with ovulation to maximize chances of fertilization.

Fallopian tubes. **Sexually transmitted infections (STIs)** can damage the lining of the fallopian tube and lead to infertility or ectopic pregnancy. A common STI is chlamydia, which often has no symptoms.

Uterus. Each month, the uterine lining prepares for a fertilized egg to implant. If a pregnancy does not occur, the ovary undergoes hormonal changes (a decrease in progesterone), which results in a menstrual period. **Fibroids** are growths of tissue in the uterine *wall*, which create an enlarged uterus. This can interfere with implantation or can even cause a miscarriage. **Polyps** are growths of tissue in the uterine *lining*, which may interfere with fertilized egg implantation (see chapter 11). Another common problem with infertility is **endometriosis** (see chapter 9).

Other Factors

Body weight may affect ovulation, resulting in irregular periods or no periods. Women who are diagnosed with anorexia or are significantly underweight may not have periods. Obesity may predispose a woman to develop high blood pressure or diabetes during pregnancy.

Excessive caffeine consumption of 200 milligrams or more a day can affect fertility. It's best not to consume more than two 6- to 8-ounce cups of coffee or other beverages that contain caffeine (such as tea, soda, or energy drinks) if you are trying to get pregnant.

Smoking is harmful to the ovaries because nicotine can affect estrogen production. This can interfere with ovulation and blood flow to the uterus, affecting the ability of the embryo to implant on the uterine lining. The effects appear to reverse soon after a woman stops smoking.

Using marijuana on a regular basis has been associated with infertility in both men and women.

Medical Conditions

Chronic conditions such as diabetes, liver, and kidney disease can affect fertility in both men and women and can affect a woman's ability to carry a pregnancy to term.

Autoimmune disorders such as thyroiditis (Hashimoto's thyroiditis), lupus, rheumatoid arthritis, celiac disease, and ulcerative colitis can affect a woman's fertility. The inflammatory processes that result from these diseases may also affect the uterine lining and possibly the placenta. Celiac disease can influence the ability to get pregnant, especially when a person has active flare-ups.

Asherman syndrome is scarring of the uterine lining that may result from a previous dilation and curettage (D&C) procedure after a miscarriage or a delivery.

Premature ovarian insufficiency is when the ovaries no longer produce or store eggs, and the patient no longer has menstrual cycles. There may be a genetic cause for this, such as Fragile X syndrome.

Sexual dysfunction is detailed in chapter 7.

Note: Talk to your health care provider about whether other medical conditions may be interfering with your ability to become pregnant.

Age

Age is associated with a decreased egg supply and poorer-quality eggs for fertilization. As you get older, especially after the age of 35, this process escalates, and it may be more difficult to become pregnant.

Unexplained Infertility

Unexplained infertility means that, after completing extensive testing, no specific cause could be identified. This is truly the most frustrating diagnosis for a patient. If you experience unexplained infertility after undergoing other treatments, it may be time to consider in vitro fertilization (IVF).

Men can experience infertility, too; for more on male infertility, see chapter 4.

Okay, I Want to Get Pregnant but Have Been Unable to Do So. What Should I Do?

Before trying to get pregnant, it is best to discuss your medical conditions, family history, and lifestyle with your health care provider. At your first office visit, your health care professional will gather a comprehensive history and may give you a physical exam. They will then discuss evaluating you and your partner for infertility and potential treatments. Part of this evaluation will involve conducting certain tests.

If it is determined that you or your partner has a fertility problem, your health care provider will work with you to develop a treatment plan.

Infertility Evaluation

At your initial infertility evaluation, your health care provider will conduct one or more of the following tests.

- Ovulation evaluation
- Ovarian reserve testing, which checks your egg supply
- Blood tests to check for anti-Mullerian hormone (AMH), **follicle-stimulating hormone (FSH)**, **luteinizing hormone (LH)**, and estradiol (E2); these tests may need to be repeated a few times for accuracy
- Fallopian tube evaluation (hysterosalpingogram or ultrasound-air fluid injection)
- Uterus and uterine cavity evaluation (ultrasound)
- Thyroid evaluation (blood tests to check serum TSH, or thyroid-stimulating hormone, and free thyroxin, or T4, levels)
- Blood tests to evaluate your immunity to German measles (rubella)
- Sperm count

Additional Tests

Depending on your individualized assessment, your health care provider may order additional blood tests to screen for cystic fibrosis, spinal muscle atrophy (SMA), and other genetic problems such as Fragile X syndrome and sickle cell disease. Depending on the circumstances, you may also need an Ashkenazi Jewish genetic panel or screening for Tay-Sachs disease, Bloom syndrome, Canavan disease, Gaucher disease, and Niemann-Pick disease.

A laparoscopy may be performed to determine the presence of endometriosis. This procedure involves the insertion of a fiberoptic instrument into the abdomen.

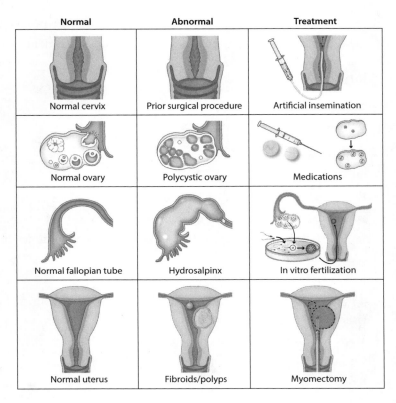

Normal	Abnormal	Treatment
Normal cervix	Prior surgical procedure	Artificial insemination
Normal ovary	Polycystic ovary	Medications
Normal fallopian tube	Hydrosalpinx	In vitro fertilization
Normal uterus	Fibroids/polyps	Myomectomy

FIGURE 3.2.

Normal and abnormal reproductive tract anatomy with corresponding treatment options.

Treatment of Common Causes of Female Infertility

Your treatment plan will be based on the type of infertility you are experiencing as well as the organs involved and the role of any medical conditions. The normal and abnormal aspects of the reproductive tract along with corresponding treatment methods are shown in figure 3.2.

Cervix

If your cervix is suspected to be the cause of your infertility, you may need **intrauterine insemination (IUI)** to become pregnant. In intrauterine insemination, a semen sample is processed to concentrate the most viable sperm and deliver them through the cervix to the uterus.

Ovaries

Ovarian disorders can be treated in a few ways to help achieve pregnancy. **Oral medications** such as **clomiphene citrate (Clomid)** and **letrozole** induce ovulation. These medications have different mechanisms of action that increase hormonal stimulation of the ovaries (from the pituitary gland) and facilitate ovulation.

Injectable medications are another option and require daily administration of FSH or HMG (human menopausal gonadotropin), which provides direct stimulation of the ovaries to develop follicles that result in ovulation.

Fallopian Tubes

Tubal damage can cause infertility and is most often treated with IVF, which is discussed in chapter 10. Your health care professional may also recommend surgery to repair the damage.

Uterus

Uterine **fibroids** are best removed with a surgical procedure called a myomectomy. A myomectomy can be performed using different surgical techniques such as hysteroscopic, laparoscopic, robotic, or open approaches. You will want to discuss with your surgeon which option is best for you.

Uterine **polyps** may interfere with implantation; operative hysteroscopy is advised for removal of the polyps. Hysteroscopy is the inspection of the uterine cavity by endoscopy with access through the cervix. It allows for the diagnosis of intrauterine pathology and serves as a method for surgical intervention.

Rare Conditions

Premature ovarian insufficiency (sometimes referred to as "early menopause") often necessitates the use of donor eggs or donor embryos in order to become pregnant.

Asherman syndrome requires surgical removal of scar tissue in the uterus, usually with operative hysteroscopy. Supplementation of the hormone estrogen is frequently prescribed after surgery.

Other medical conditions and autoimmune disorders require specialized treatment. Your health care provider will work with you on an individualized treatment plan based on your specific needs.

Unexplained infertility treatment options vary. Some doctors prescribe medications such as Clomid or letrozole, often with IUI, or they may suggest timed intercourse. More aggressive treatment includes the addition of other medications administered by injection to trigger ovulation. If these steps are not successful, IVF may be required.

Anjali's Story

I HAVE BEEN A TEACHER for a long time, and being surrounded by school-aged children has finally convinced me that I want a child. My husband and I have been married for five years, and once we agreed that we were ready to have a family, I felt it was important to see my gynecologist. My nurse practitioner mentioned that this first appointment would be called the "preconception counseling visit," which sounds about right to me!

After counseling on ovulation predictor kits, we embarked on this journey. While it was fun at the beginning, the process quickly became a depressing chore. Every time I got my period, I started to feel irritated and angry. After six months, I called my gynecologist, who kindly encouraged me and advised that since I was only 30, I should keep trying for at least a year.

Unfortunately, a year and a half later, I went back to my gynecologist with no new updates. She suggested I see an infertility specialist, which while disheartening to hear, still gave me a hopeful step forward. At my first appointment, the doctor asked both my husband and me several questions and suggested a number of tests. One week later, he called me back to discuss my results. I had a "unicornuate uterus." What does that mean?

He explained that my uterus did not fully form during fetal development, leaving me with half of a functioning uterus and making it difficult to carry a pregnancy to full term. To my dismay, I also learned that there is a higher chance of having preeclampsia, or high blood pressure, with my abnormal uterus.

My husband and I grieved over the situation but then talked to the infertility specialist again and decided upon IVF. The specialist suggested that we genetically test the embryos ahead of time. We completed round one, and unfortunately all the embryos had abnormalities . . . of course this happened to us. We've decided to give the IVF process one more go—please send us some luck!

• TAKEAWAY POINTS •

Women under the age of 35 trying for one year and women age 35 or older trying for six months or more to become pregnant are considered to have female infertility.

If you are 40 or older and wish to become pregnant, you should seek an evaluation by an infertility specialist. Check out the website of the American Society for Reproductive Medicine to find specialists in your area (www.reproductivefacts.org).

Women experience an age-related decline in egg supply starting at age 35.

There are multiple causes of infertility, including ones that occur only in men.

When planning for pregnancy, a preconception counseling visit is recommended.

The sooner you seek care, the better.

Infertility treatment depends on the cause.

Unexplained infertility can also be treated.

• KEY WORDS •

clomiphene citrate (Clomid)
follicle-stimulating hormone (FSH)
intrauterine insemination (IUI)
letrozole (off-label use)
luteinizing hormone (LH)
ovulation

Chapter 4

We're Part of It, Too

Male Infertility

THE CALL FROM THE DOCTOR'S office came at 9 a.m. today, and I have been sitting in my chair for the past 45 minutes trying to make sense of what I just learned. The results of my semen analysis test from earlier in the week just came in, and I was told that my sperm count is very low. How could that happen? I mean . . . I have never even thought about such a possibility. I am so embarrassed. The doctor's office wants me to come in so I can discuss this condition with him in detail. I don't know how I am going to tell Svetlana about this. She will be so stressed, especially since we have been trying to get pregnant for the past couple months.—*Ivan*

What You Need to Know about Male Infertility

How Common Is It? Is It Easy to Fix?

From a statistical perspective, male infertility is seen in 40% to 50% of infertile couples. Overall, male infertility affects 7% of all men. The causes of male infertility can be problems with semen volume, sperm count, movement, or motility as well as shapes of the sperm.

TABLE 4.1.
Characteristics of a semen analysis

PARAMETERS	NORMAL VALUES
Volume (seminal fluid)	1.5 mL or more
Count	≥15 million/mL sperm
Motility (movement)	32% or more
Normal shapes (morphology)	4% or greater

If your health care provider suspects that male infertility is involved with your difficulties getting pregnant, a **semen analysis** may be performed. This analysis will help determine whether there are any of the above problems with the sperm. Several benchmarks are used to evaluate whether the semen is "normal," including the Kruger criteria and criteria from the World Health Organization (WHO). The parameters involved with a semen analysis, as well as what values are considered to be in the normal range, are listed in table 4.1.

How Do They Count Sperm? What's a Good Number? Can You Have Too Many?

When obtaining a semen sample, it is best to abstain from sex for several (2–10) days and avoid drinking alcohol. Care must be taken to obtain the complete specimen and have it processed promptly. Some urologists prefer more than one sample to get a broader evaluation of a man's fertility. **Urologists** are trained to examine and evaluate male anatomy, which includes the penis, testicles, and remainder of the male reproductive tract. A physical examination is usually followed by blood tests to measure testosterone as well as the pituitary gland hormones. Additional tests, such as imaging (ultrasound) of the scrotal area, may be recommended.

What Are the Terms That Describe an Abnormal Semen Analysis?

If your semen analysis indicates problems with your sperm, you may see the terms azoospermia, oligospermia, asthenospermia, asthenozoosper-

TABLE 4.2.
Terms used to describe findings in a semen analysis

TERM	CLINICAL DEFINITION
Azoospermia	No sperm
Oligospermia	Decreased number of sperm
Asthenospermia or asthenozoospermia	Decreased motility (movement)
Teratozoospermia	Abnormal sperm shapes

mia, or teratozoospermia. These terms are defined in table 4.2. Pictographic representations of these problems appear in figure 4.1.

What Are the Causes of Male Infertility?

Male infertility can be attributed to a number of risk factors (figure 4.2).

Anatomic causes of male infertility include a varicocele, which is a swelling of veins in the scrotum; testicular torsion, or twisting; and rarely mumps orchitis, hydrocele, and vas deferens (tubing) defects. Hypogonadism is when the pituitary gland does not produce adequate hormones (follicle-stimulating hormone and luteinizing hormone) to stimulate the testes. Undescended testes is a condition in which the testes do not go down into the scrotal sacs.

Medications can interfere with fertility; discuss any medications you are taking with your health care provider.

Environmental causes of infertility include smoking, vaping, marijuana use, alcohol consumption, and taking illicit drugs.

Hormones can play a role; your health care provider may order tests of your hormone levels and thyroid function.

Genetic problems such as Klinefelter syndrome and cryptorchidism (undescended testicle) can lead to infertility.

Athletic activities may affect a man's fertility. Strenuous exercise such as excessive cycling or horseback riding can lower sperm count or cause some of the anatomical problems listed above.

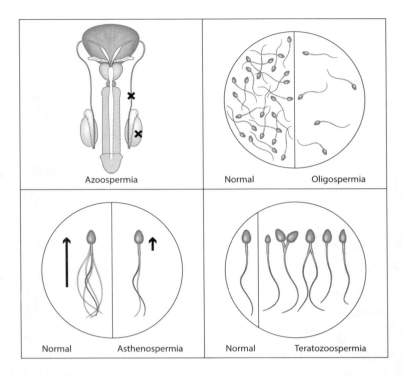

FIGURE 4.1.
Types of male infertility, including examples of normal versus abnormal sperm.

Anatomical Causes

One of the more common causes of male infertility is a varicocele, or varicose veins around the testicle. On examination, it is described as feeling like a "bag of worms" when the area is palpated (figure 4.3). Varicocele affects 15% of fertile males and 40% of infertile males.

A testicle can twist, termed torsion. Testicle torsion has a negative effect on sperm production. It most often is associated with pain in the testicles.

Fluid around the testes is a condition called hydrocele.

Other causes of male infertility are mumps involving the testicles (what is known as mumps orchitis) and trauma to the testes. Men who produce no sperm (a condition called azoospermia) may be missing a

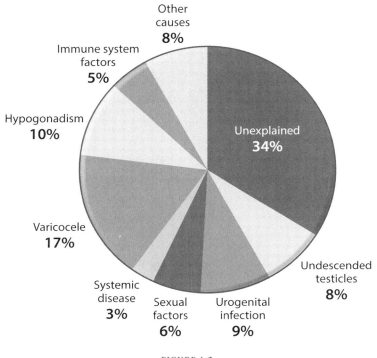

FIGURE 4.2.
Causes of male infertility.

portion of the tube that runs from the testicle (the vas deferens), a rare occurrence. A male may also have vas obstruction, which is when the vas deferens is blocked. This blockage acts much like a vasectomy, which is performed for sterilization and involves the deliberate interference of the tubing leaving the testicle. On occasion, the sperm cannot penetrate the egg to result in fertilization; this may be due to abnormality involving the sperm head, termed acrosomal defects.

Medications

Testosterone therapy can result in a low sperm count. In addition, certain antibiotics, some ulcer medications, and antifungal medications can

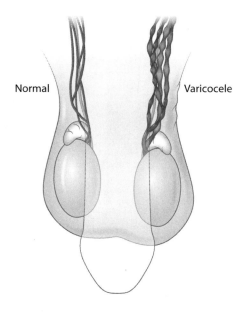

Normal
Varicocele

FIGURE 4.3.
Male reproductive tract abnormality: varicocele.

cause a low sperm count. Make sure to discuss any medications you are taking with your doctor.

Environmental Factors

Other causes of infertility include smoking or vaping, as tobacco smoke can damage sperm production. Additionally, smoking increases intake of cadmium, which affects zinc levels that influence DNA (deoxyribonucleic acid) activity, and thus poor sperm production results. Marijuana can affect sperm production and possibly affect chromosomes. Alcohol, especially in excessive amounts, and illicit drugs also have adverse effects on sperm.

Hormonal Factors

Hormonal problems can occur at the brain-pituitary level, with the result that the testes do not receive the hormones to stimulate production of sperm. Thyroid disorders such as hypothyroidism and hyperthyroidism can also affect sperm production. Obesity can be associated with a decrease in sperm count.

Genetic Factors

Genetic disorders that cause azoospermia are sometimes, although rarely, the cause. Failure of the testes to descend into the scrotum, called cryptorchidism, affects sperm production. Sometimes there is no apparent cause for lack of sperm, which is termed idiopathic failure. An unexplained decrease in sperm count is called idiopathic oligospermia. Tumors growing inside the testicle can affect sperm production. The most common tumor (also known as a neoplasm) is a seminoma.

Klinefelter syndrome is a rare disorder that may lead to male infertility. Males with Klinefelter syndrome have 47 chromosomes XXY instead of the 46 XY in men who do not have the disorder. The syndrome is associated with low testosterone levels, tall stature, fat depositions in the abdomen, coordination problems, and lower muscle strength. These men may have smaller testes and penis, breast development (gynecomastia), less facial and body hair, weaker bones, decreased libido, and reduced sperm production. Should a diagnosis of Klinefelter syndrome be made, it may be wise to save (bank) sperm early on, meaning soon after onset of puberty.

Other Causes

Various other problems can lead to male infertility, including inflammation of the prostate, termed prostatitis. Pain around the penis, testicles, or lower abdomen, especially when urinating, may indicate prostatitis. Another symptom of prostatitis is urgency, where you feel the need to urinate but no or minimal urine comes out. Prostatitis can also be associated with blood in urine (hematuria).

On rare occasion, the penile opening is not at the end of the penis but along the shaft. This condition, called hypospadias, can be surgically corrected. Lastly, retrograde ejaculation can occur when the sperm at the time of ejaculation go into the bladder and not out the penis.

I Have a Normal Sperm Count. What Else Could Be Wrong with Me?

Male infertility can be related to sexual dysfunction, where a man has decreased libido or is not able to achieve or maintain an erection. This condition, known as **erectile dysfunction** or **impotence**, has a number of causes. Diseases like diabetes can affect the nerves in the penis, leading to a condition called diabetic neuropathy, which can cause erectile dysfunction. Prior surgery in the area of the testes, such as a hernia repair, could affect or disrupt the nerves, blood supply, or "tubing." Impotence can have a psychological cause and is best dealt with by a professional with mental health expertise.

What Are the Options to Treat Male Fertility?

There are both medical and surgical treatment options, which your health care provider should discuss with you. You may need medications, hormone therapy, or surgery. Your provider may also refer you to a urologist for further evaluation and treatment.

Medications

Your doctor may prescribe clomiphene citrate (Clomid) to increase your sperm count. If your infertility has a hormonal cause, pituitary gland hormone injections may be indicated. Inflammatory conditions such as prostatitis are treated with antibiotics and/or antisteroidals.

Surgical Options

Depending on the diagnosis, surgery by a urologist may be necessary. If a man has no sperm upon semen analysis, it may be possible to extract sperm directly from the testicle, a procedure called **testicular sperm extraction (TESE)**. The sperm can be extracted in a variety of ways. Testicular sperm extraction virtually always requires in vitro fertilization (IVF) to achieve a pregnancy. In this process, one sperm is injected into one egg (ICSI, or intracytoplasmic sperm injection). For men who experience ejaculation into the bladder (retrograde ejaculation), a urologist may be able to treat their condition medically.

Lifestyle Changes

One or more lifestyle changes may help treat male infertility. Below are some ways you may be able to take charge of your fertility.

- Eat a healthy diet and exercise regularly.
- Lose weight if you are obese.
- Avoid saunas, hot tubs, and hot showers.
- Take a multivitamin that contains zinc.
- Try to minimize stress.
- Address any existing medical problems.
- Discuss your medications with the prescribing doctor, and ask whether they affect sperm count.
- Avoid alcohol and illicit drugs.
- Stop smoking or vaping.
- Get adequate sleep.
- Avoid placing laptops and other electronics in your lap, as these can increase the temperature in the scrotal region.
- Consider wearing boxer shorts that allow the testicle to be further from the body compared to tight-fitting underwear.

Chris's Story

I READ THAT YOU SHOULD HAVE sex three days in a row mid-cycle, and we did this month after month after deciding to start a family. Lauren was faithfully taking prenatal vitamins, always careful about her "lifestyle," diet, exercise, and would only take an occasional drink.

I have always been a go-getter and have successfully run a business in automotive repair. I have always been good about my lifestyle—never smoking, trying to work out three times a week, keeping beer for the weekends, and maintaining excellent health.

We proceeded with the infertility work-up, and everything checked out okay for Lauren. But when I got a semen analysis, I was shocked to find out I had "no sperm." Now I have to sit down with the doctor and discuss the results. I am not sure I want to do this. The doctor went through each test result for Lauren. He said, "Your tubes are open, the cavity of your uterus looks fine, the egg supply is good, thyroid is normal, no signs of cystic fibrosis or other things, you are not a carrier." Lauren sighed with relief.

Then he turned to me and said, "Chris, I reviewed your semen analysis, and there was no sperm." I felt my face flush a deep beet red. From that moment, I tuned out everything else he said. Lauren looked at me and the doctor, horrified. I knew she was thinking we might never have a baby, and in that moment I felt a deep sense of guilt. The doctor recommended that I repeat the semen analysis and see a male infertility-urologist specialist.

As advised by our doctor, I went to the urologist, who took detailed information about my medical history and examined me. She said in part she was looking for a problem around the testicles. The exam was normal. The urologist sent my doctor a report following her evaluation. She checked my hormones and concluded that my testosterone was low and the hormones from the pituitary gland stimulating the testes were high. A testicular biopsy showed no sperm. She assured me that I was not alone and that other men have had similar test results.

After much introspection and discussion, Lauren and I elected to proceed with donor inseminations. We timed the insemination with medicine to enhance ovulation, using one injection to trigger ovulation and do the insemination within 36 hours.

We proceeded with cycle 1 but no pregnancy. With cycle 2 we were disappointed again. Finally, with cycle 3 we got a positive pregnancy test. We were elated. I often look at my now-teenage son and am so thankful for the opportunity to be a father.

• TAKEAWAY POINTS •

Infertility affects 7% of all men.

As many as 40% to 50% of couples have a "male factor" when it comes to infertility.

Evaluation is best done by a urologist, ideally one trained in male infertility.

Many factors can cause male infertility.

Semen analysis collection must be done properly and evaluated by a lab professional.

Varicocele can be associated with infertility.

Testicular torsion is associated with testicle pain.

Pregnancy is possible with in vitro fertilization with no sperm in the ejaculate if sperm can be extracted from the testicle.

• KEY WORDS •

impotence / erectile dysfunction
semen analysis
testicular sperm extraction (TESE)
urologist

Chapter 5

The Embryo Just Won't Stick

Reproductive Immunology

ALEX AND I HAVE BEEN MARRIED for only two years, but we decided early that we did not want to wait too long to begin a family. Excited and full of hope, we decided to use an ovulation predictor kit to time sex. I was elated when my pregnancy test came back positive. However, two weeks later, I had a heavy period, and that was it for that pregnancy.

Time passed, and I decided we need to try again. Everything was the same, but this time the blood HCG (human chorionic gonadotropin) level doubled in two days! Alex and I got to hear our baby's heartbeat for the first time, and I cried with joy. Two weeks after the ultrasound, though, I began vaginal bleeding, spotting at first, then heavy. I went back for an ultrasound. The heartbeat was no longer there, and my doctor said, "I am sorry, but you had an embryonic demise." She said that we could either take medications to expel the pregnancy or proceed with a dilation and curettage. I chose the D&C. Time progressed, and I had enough courage to try again. Unfortu-

nately, we had the same result—an ultrasound with a heartbeat, bleeding, and miscarriage. Why do my pregnancies end
up like this?

My doctor said, "While we don't have all the answers, let
me answer your question why like this. Most of the time, a miscarriage is because the embryo is genetically abnormal." She
also said, "We know there is 'cross-talk' between the embryo
and the lining of your uterus. In some women, the uterus rejects the pregnancy, and this is what we term an 'immunologic
cause' for miscarriages."—*Malia*

What You Need to Know about Pregnancy Loss

Chemical Pregnancy

Pregnancies are considered to be "chemical" if the only evidence is
a positive blood test. A **chemical pregnancy**, which happens primarily
in the first trimester, is a type of very early miscarriage.

What Is Recurrent Pregnancy Loss?

Recurrent pregnancy loss is defined as two or more miscarriages per the
American College of Obstetricians and Gynecologists (ACOG).

Evaluation for Recurrent Pregnancy Loss

If you have had two or more miscarriages, your health care provider
may do additional examinations or tests to determine what is causing
the pregnancy loss, including:

- Anatomic examination of the uterus by ultrasound
- Endocrinology (hormone) evaluation
- Thyroid testing
- Blood sugar (can be hemoglobin A1c)

- Check of the progesterone level during the second half of your menstrual cycle
- Immunologic blood tests
- Test for presence of Beta 2-glycoprotein
- Anticardiolipin antibodies (ACA)
- Genetic (karyotyping) of you and your partner
- Assessment of the male partner's fertility status

Who Should Be Evaluated for Recurrent Pregnancy Loss?

Anyone who has a history of the following should seek an evaluation.

- Two or more miscarriages
- Immunologic diagnosis:
  - rheumatoid arthritis
  - lupus
  - Hashimoto's thyroiditis
  - celiac disease
  - other immunologic disorders
- Poor egg quality and embryo development
- Abnormal fetal growth in a prior pregnancy
- Recurrent miscarriages after in vitro fertilization

Reproductive Immunology

The immune system plays a key role in pregnancy establishment and maintenance. Researchers believe there is "cross-talk" between the embryo and the uterine lining. An embryo that does not have genetic defects tends to implant more readily than a chromosomally abnormal embryo. An image of normal implantation in the lining of the uterus is shown in figure 5.1. Most miscarriages are due to abnormal embryo genetics.

Reproductive immunology is a field that focuses on the interplay between the immune system and the reproductive system. A woman who has recurrent miscarriages may have an immune response that con-

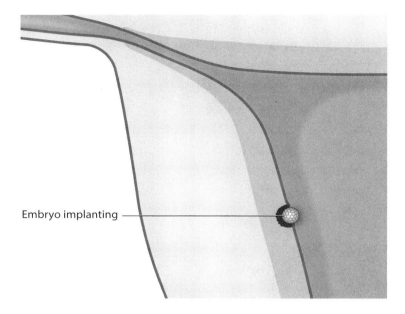

Embryo implanting

FIGURE 5.1.
Embryo implanting in the uterus.

siders the embryo trying to implant as an "invader" and rejects it from implanting. This is known as immunologic infertility. The body's immune response may also be responsible for premature birth and preeclampsia (high blood pressure during pregnancy). Treatment focuses on reducing the inflammation and suppressing the immune system, allowing for successful implantation and pregnancy.

Tests for Immunologic Infertility

If your health care provider suspects that an immunologic response is the reason for your infertility, they may order a test for one or more of the following.

- Antinuclear antibodies (ANA)
- Antiphospholipid antibodies

- Beta 2-glycoprotein
- Antithyroid antibodies
- Natural killer cell assay
- Helper T1 and T2 assay
- Regulatory T cells
- Reproductive immunophenotypes CD-3, CD-4, CD-8, CD-5, CD-16, CD-19, and CD-56, associated with thrombophilia (blood clots)

Some of these tests remain at the research level.

Treatment for Immunologic Infertility

Because research in the field of reproductive immunology is ongoing, the treatment of immunologic infertility varies and is somewhat unproven. Some studies recommend low-dose steroids such as prednisone and low-dose (81-milligram) aspirin. Intralipids and intravenous immunoglobulins are sometimes administered to suppress the immune system's response to in vitro fertilization (IVF). Until well-designed studies are available, these treatments remain controversial.

Dietary changes may help treat immunological problems, such as avoiding excessive amounts of carbohydrates, refined sugars, and dairy products, but here again what is lacking are well-designed, randomized controlled trials (RCTs). Having someone carry your genetic embryo (what is called a gestational carrier or surrogate) is an option, but again we lack good studies to advise this approach.

Malala's Story

I AM TOTALLY FRUSTRATED. I have been pregnant four times, and none have gone beyond three months. Now my male partner and I are afraid to even try to get pregnant. I am 38 years old and have no kids. I used to have painful periods, but they have been tolerable ever since my very first pregnancy. I have suffered from anxiety and depression, but taking my meds keeps those conditions well controlled. When I cough or sneeze, I lose a little bit of urine; I've had that checked out by a urogynecologist, and they have me do Kegel exercises when I pee. That seems to correct the problem. I was told I have endometriosis, but surgery is required for a definitive diagnosis, and I'm not up for that. I searched the Internet and found a reproductive immunologist, and I think that she might be able to help me.

I told the doctor my story and as many details as I could remember about each of the pregnancies. During my last pregnancy, we did chromosome studies, and it was a normal female. The doctor took the time to explain each test I would need going forward, including testing of a variety of antibodies and genetic testing.

Wow, it felt like they took a gallon of blood for the tests. We went back after all the tests were done, and the doctor suggested I be placed on heparin and prednisone as soon as I have a positive pregnancy test. She also talked about other treatment like baby aspirin daily and intravenous immunoglobulins but said the best treatment is the heparin and the other two medications.

Somewhat overwhelmed, we drove back home, talked about it, and decided we would try for another pregnancy. We went back to our local infertility doctor. Got pregnant and started the heparin and prednisone. We actually made it into the second trimester, meaning we made it beyond three months. I so much looked forward to each OB-GYN visit, listening to the baby's heart. They checked my blood sugar, and then I had to drink this yucky stuff to test my glucose. The test result showed I had gestational diabetes and needed to control it with diet. Honestly, I will do everything the doctors and nurses tell me to do for this pregnancy. Time progressed and we entered the third trimester—the home stretch. We are wary but very hopeful for an outcome that we have been waiting for years.

• TAKEAWAY POINTS •

Two or more miscarriages warrant evaluation by a fertility specialist.

An evaluation of pregnancy loss should include examination of the uterine cavity, a check of hormonal (endocrinologic) function, immunologic testing, and an assessment of the couple's genetics.

Treatment of immunologic infertility is controversial but can include steroids such as prednisone and low-dose aspirin.

• KEY WORDS •

chemical pregnancy
recurrent pregnancy loss
reproductive immunology

Chapter 6

Not Tonight, Wait till Ovulation

Sexual Dysfunction

TODAY IS NOT JUST ANOTHER DAY at the pizza shop. My wife told me there was something serious she wanted to talk about. I know that things have been tense at home; we've been trying to have a child for the past two years. The worst part is that I feel like it is my fault. Jess is a healthy woman and we've used all the ovulation predictor kits, but I cannot always get an erection, and the frustration escalates for both of us. Jess just told me that she wants me to come to see the OB-GYN with her. Why would I do that? Could there really be something wrong with me? Does this make me less of a man?—*Michael*

What You Need to Know about Sexual Dysfunction

Is Something Wrong with Me?

Sexual dysfunction affects both men and women. The **sexual response** has four phases (American College of Obstetricians and Gynecologists,

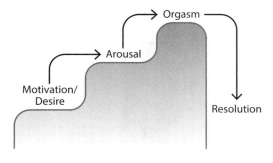

FIGURE 6.1.
Segments of the sex cycle.

2019), any one of which can be involved with sexual dysfunction (figure 6.1).

1. Desire (libido)
2. Arousal (excitement)
3. Orgasm
4. Resolution

Desire is usually at least partly a reflection of the relationship and communication between the couple. There are multiple factors that can make sex less desirable. Pain experienced by the woman during intercourse can be a symptom of endometriosis or prior pelvic infection. Stress, depression, anxiety medications, neurologic problems, and substance use can also contribute to sexual dysfunction, for both men and women. Alcohol can have a negative effect on a couple's sex life. It can affect a man's ability to get and maintain an erection. As a depressant, alcohol can diminish the mood. It can also interfere with the ability to have an orgasm.

During the excitement phase, there is increased blood flow to the vagina, and the clitoris becomes more sensitive. Men also experience increased blood flow to the penis during the excitement phase, which results in an erection.

Orgasm for both men and women is associated with involuntary muscle contractions, increase in blood pressure and heart rate, and a forceful release of sexual tension.

During resolution, both partners' bodies slowly return to a baseline level of functioning; in other words, this is the "recovery" phase.

We would be remiss if we didn't acknowledge the work of William H. Masters, Virginia E. Johnson, and Helen Singer Kaplan when it comes to our understanding of sexual function and dysfunction. Masters and Johnson were part of the Kinsey Institute. They conducted pioneering studies on the nature of the human sexual response. Helen Singer Kaplan described three stages of the sexual response: desire, excitement, and orgasm. The work of these researchers was in the 1960s and remains an integral part of what we know today. As one researcher aptly stated, they "brought science to the bedroom" ("Pioneering 'Masters,'" 2013).

What Are the Types of Female Sexual Dysfunction?

The *Diagnostic and Statistical Manual of Mental Disorders* (American Psychiatric Association, 2013) describes several types of **female sexual dysfunction**.

- Female sexual interest/arousal disorder
- Female orgasmic disorder
- Pelvic pain/penetration disorder (vaginismus)
- Substance- or medication-induced sexual dysfunction
- Other specified or unspecified sexual dysfunction

Orgasmic disorders can be lifelong (primary anorgasmia) or acquired. There is a distinction between clitoral orgasm and vaginal orgasm. The former is a normal variation to the sexual response. At least one-third of all women do not experience vaginal orgasm. Situational factors can also account for acquired lack of orgasm.

Painful intercourse (dyspareunia) can have a number of causes. It can be due to endometriosis or scar tissue in the pelvic organs. Scarring can

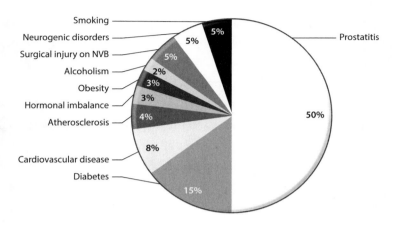

FIGURE 6.2.
The underlying causes of erectile dysfunction. NVB, neurovascular bundle.

be caused by a sexually transmitted infection, or it can be the result of a medical procedure. Pain during sex can have psychological causes, too. Vulvar pain (vulvodynia) is a separate type of female sexual pain disorder.

If you have symptoms of sexual dysfunction, your health care provider can assess your sexual function, desire, lubrication, pain, and ability to have orgasms. They may use a questionnaire such as the Patient-Reported Outcomes Measurement Information System to help identify sexual problems. The provider may perform a pelvic examination for more information, especially if you have pain with intercourse. You may want to consult a mental health professional if you suspect there are psychological causes.

What about Male Sexual Dysfunction?

Men experience sexual dysfunction, too, most often in the form of **erectile dysfunction** (figure 6.2). There are numerous causes that range from psychological to medical to decreased blood flow to the penis. Premature ejaculation, while it lacks a hard and fast definition, is generally considered to be an orgasm that occurs within two minutes from the time of penile insertion. This, too, can be a problem for a couple. **Male sexual dysfunction** is best evaluated by a urologist and possibly a sex therapist as well. Treatment depends on the cause. Medications such as Viagra, Cialis, Levitra, and Stendra are prescribed to dilate blood vessels and allow an erection. Penile injections such as Alprostadil can be injected directly into the shaft of the penis to cause an erection. Psychological causes may need to be addressed by a mental health professional. Smoking, alcohol, and low testosterone have also been implicated with erectile dysfunction. It is best to have a health care professional evaluate the problem and order treatment accordingly.

What Questions Might Be Asked When Evaluating Sexual Dysfunction?

It's normal to feel nervous or uncomfortable about discussing sexual dysfunction with your doctor. But your answers to their questions will help your health care provider create a treatment plan for you and your partner. Below are some examples of the questions they might ask you (Kingsberg et al., 2017).

- How long has this been a problem?
- What was happening in your life when it began?
- How often do you initiate sexual activity?
- How often do you have sexual relations?
- Are there circumstances in which you are not interested in sex?
- Is there "mental excitement" during intercourse?
- Do you have pain?
- How often do you have an orgasm?
- How much of a problem is low sexual desire for you?
- Are you happy with your relationship?
- Does your partner have sexual problems?
- Rate your level of interest in sex (0 to 10, with 10 being the highest).
- What are you looking for from treatment?

ι Be Treated?

ices, and other therapies may be indicated to treat sex-
~~ual~~ dysfunction depending on the cause. Your health care provider is the
best source to determine what treatment is best for you.

Medications

Medications for sexual dysfunction include:

- DHEA (dehydroepiandrosterone) for erectile dysfunction
- Duloxetine (trade name Cymbalta) for anxiety
- Flibanserin for hypoactive sexual desire disorder
- Sildenafil citrate (Viagra) for erectile dysfunction
- Bupropion for depression
- Buspirone (Wellbutrin, Zyban) for depression
- Lybrido/Lybridos for hypoactive sexual desire disorder
- Mirtazapine (Remeron) for depression
- Tibolone for postmenopausal women

Innovative Devices

In some cases, bringing a device into the bedroom can help treat sexual
dysfunction in men and women. Battery-powered clitoral suction devices
such as the Eros are designed to improve arousal and blood flow to the
clitoris. For men, erectile dysfunction devices such as Encore and, depending on the circumstances, penile pumps (also known as a penile prosthe-
sis) can be placed by a urologist. The patient can then control the pump
manually before having sex.

Patient Education

Perhaps at the top of the list for treatment is patient education. Let's begin with hypoactive sexual desire, which is far and away the most common problem. Both men and women can experience hypoactive sexual

desire, which is defined as a lack of arousal or interest in sex or sexual fantasy. Because sexual desire involves many factors, there could be more than one cause of the lack of interest in sex. Your health care provider should explore psychological factors such as depression, as well as any medications you are taking. The relationship you have with your partner, changes in your life, and your motivation for engaging in sexual intercourse are but a few of the aspects of assessment and treatment. An effort to identify the underlying problem or precipitating factors is most important. Your health care professional will help determine the underlying cause and treat it accordingly.

Psychologists and other allied health professionals are trained to treat sexual dysfunction. When looking for help in this area, you should seek a provider who is a member of the Society for Sex Therapy and Research (SSTAR), the American Association of Sexuality Educators (AASECT), or one of the other groups listed in the Resources section (page 197). Orgasm-related problems can be addressed by individuals with sexual skills training. You may be able to improve your sexual functioning by enhancing communication with your partner. Group-based therapy may also be a good option for treatment.

Other Treatments

In addition to the therapies outlined above, the following treatments may help.

- Cognitive behavioral therapy, or CBT, focuses on identifying the cause of sexual dysfunction and helping the patient learn mental strategies to work through the problem.
- Stress management may be a key to success.
- If vaginal penetration is the problem, vaginal dilators may be useful.
- Physical therapy of the pelvic floor can improve the vaginal and rectal musculature; biofeedback may also be of assistance.

- Adequate lubrication may be all that is needed to make sex more enjoyable and successful. Be sure to choose a vaginal lubricant that does not affect sperm survival, such as one of the following:
  - Astroglide
  - Pre-Seed
  - Baby Dance
  - Food-grade oils (coconut, olive, and vegetable)

Trish's Story

I AM 31 YEARS OLD, have been married for six years, and love my husband. I am a stay-at-home mom and love spending time with our beautiful daughter, who is 4 years old. We don't use birth control and are hoping we might have a second child. After trying for some time with no luck, we decided we should go to the doctor to see why we aren't getting pregnant.

The doctor was great—made me feel at ease. We were sitting across from each other, and as he went through a list of questions, he got to the topic of sex. He asked if we were timing sex with ovulation. Because we were wanting to make things "as spontaneous as possible," I answered no. He asked how often we had sex. I answered, "Once a week." Do you have any pain? My answer, "No." Then he asked if we have had any change in desire, and that opened a can of worms! I needed a tissue, as the tears started. My husband and I had a wonderful sex life, never a problem. We used to have sex three times a week at least before our daughter was born. But I confess that I'm not interested in sex anymore. It's so frustrating! Well, we proceeded with my providing information about my past medical history, medications, family history, and my husband did the same.

Then came the exam, which included a pelvic examination. The doctor concluded that everything looked good and that we would focus on tests regarding getting pregnant. But then he said something very important to me. "I'm not ignoring your lack of sex drive, and I am going to refer you to a psychologist that specializes in that. I think she can help you." Thank heavens, I thought to myself.

I went to see this person, and she made me feel comfortable. I won't elaborate on all the details, but she did emphasize the importance of communication with my husband. She talked about a diagnosis of "hypoactive sexual desire disorder." I went right home and Googled it. I found it is a persistent or recurrent deficiency of sexual fantasies or thoughts along with a lack of desire for or receptivity to sexual activity, all of which causes distress. It fit perfectly, including when my husband was the initiator. I would often say, "Not tonight, honey." Speaking of that, I used to have no problem with orgasms, and now it's a chore to achieve one.

The psychologist gave me a list of "Risk Factors for Hypoactive Sexual Desire Disorder." It included a lot of answers about why someone might develop the condition, including poor self-esteem, poor quality of relationship, stress, boring sexual routine, situational disturbances, depression, medical problems like diabetes, medications, and low testosterone.

She suggested we "break out of our routine" and avoid rushed bedtime encounters, which tend to be less satisfying because of time constraints and being exhausted. She said we should spend time strengthening our relationship and focus on sexual intimacy. That she was here for us and suggested a follow-up session. It's working, I think!

• TAKEAWAY POINTS •

Problems around sexual desire are the most common concerns for women struggling with sexual dysfunction.

Erectile dysfunction in men can be treated based upon the cause.

Sex therapy by trained professionals can be most rewarding.

Education for the patient and partner is an excellent place to start.

• KEY WORDS •

erectile dysfunction
female sexual dysfunction
male sexual dysfunction
sexual response

Chapter 7

No Periods for Me

Amenorrhea

I HAVE ALWAYS BEEN VERY ATHLETIC. While in high school, I ran marathons and loved to work out. I was also careful about what I ate and would always "watch my calories." I started having periods at 12, and they were irregular for a year and a half. Then, like clockwork, they came every month. I noticed that if I ran a marathon or really worked out a lot, my periods would stop. I got married and talked to my husband, John, about getting pregnant. John didn't say anything at the time, but later on he told me, "I was thinking to myself, 'If her periods are absent, since she is such a great athlete right now, how can we ever get pregnant?'" John decided to bring up the subject of getting pregnant and suggested I see a doctor about getting pregnant. Good advice indeed!—*Gillian*

What You Need to Know about Amenorrhea

Lack of periods, also termed **amenorrhea**, is not all that uncommon. The causes are many, and we will address the details. Lack of periods is classified as either primary amenorrhea (meaning when a girl has never had a period by age 14 without breast and pubic hair development, or when a girl

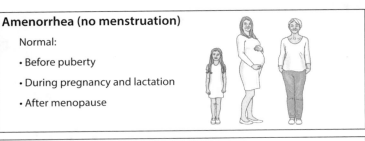

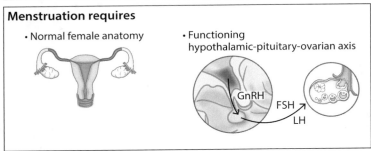

FIGURE 7.1.
Causes of amenorrhea. FSH, follicle-stimulating hormone; GnRH,
gonadotropin-releasing hormone; LH, luteinizing hormone.

has never had a period by 16 with such development) or secondary amenorrhea (when the menstrual cycle has stopped for a female who previously had periods). There is also physiologic amenorrhea, which is when periods stop because of pregnancy or breastfeeding. Menopause is associated with no periods; this includes early or premature menopause, better termed premature ovarian insufficiency.

What Causes Amenorrhea?

It is normal for a female not to menstruate if she has not yet reached puberty, she is pregnant or lactating, or is menopausal (figure 7.1).

There may be a medical or environmental reason why a woman might not menstruate, including:

- Lack of ovulation (known as anovulation)
- Premature ovarian insufficiency, or early menopause

- Stress
- Exercise-induced (athletic) amenorrhea
- Eating disorders such as anorexia and bulimia
- Increased prolactin levels (hyperprolactinemia)
- Polycystic ovarian syndrome, or PCOS
- Thyroid disorders
- Elevated male hormones, which can cause acne and facial hair
- Medication-induced amenorrhea
- Medical conditions such as hemochromatosis or celiac disease
- Uterine scarring (Asherman syndrome)

How Does Menstruation Normally Work?

Once a girl reaches puberty, signals from the brain travel to the ovaries via the bloodstream. The ovary responds by developing an egg. If no pregnancy occurs, the hormone levels drop, and the woman starts her period.

The brain controls the menstrual cycle through the pituitary gland, which makes hormones—**follicle-stimulating hormone (FSH)** and **luteinizing hormone (LH)**—that enter the bloodstream and stimulate the ovary to develop an egg. The pituitary gland receives signals (hormones) from the hypothalamus, which is located right above it. The hypothalamic hormone is **gonadotropin-releasing hormone (GnRH)**. Each month, 1,000 follicles are stimulated in the ovaries, but only one develops into an egg (occasionally it is more than one egg). In response to the pituitary hormones, the ovary makes estrogen, which enters the bloodstream and tells the pituitary gland (and hypothalamus) to slow down hormone release in response to the growing pregnancy. This process, known as the **hypothalamic-pituitary-ovarian axis**, is illustrated in figure 7.2.

Another form of amenorrhea is called **functional hypothalamic amenorrhea (FHA)**, which is characterized by a lack of FSH and LH production and release. The medical term for the result of these low hormone releases is hypogonadotropic hypogonadism, and it often occurs with

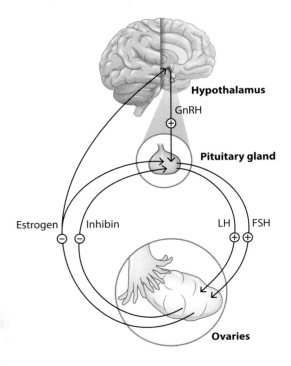

FIGURE 7.2.
Hypothalamic-pituitary-ovarian axis. FSH, follicle-stimulating hormone; GnRH, gonadotropin-releasing hormone; LH, luteinizing hormone.

anorexia and sometimes with bulimia. Women with hypogonadotropic hypogonadism have low estrogen levels and can have thinning of the bones (osteoporosis) or a milder decrease in bone mineral density (osteopenia) in addition to no periods. Some factors that influence FHA include chronic stress, overexercising, and low body mass index (BMI). We have personally observed that high achievers have FHA more frequently. In extreme cases, heart- and neurological-related problems can occur. Many times, small amounts of weight gain or decreasing the level of athletic activity corrects the problem, and the patient resumes ovulation and menstrual cycles.

There may be a genetic component to not having periods. Idiopathic hypogonadotropic hypogonadism (IHH) represents a deficiency of GnRH and thus no FSH and LH or ovarian stimulation to develop an egg. IHH appears to have a genetic basis.

What Tests Can Evaluate Amenorrhea?

If you are not having a period, your health care provider may order one or more tests to determine the cause.

- Pregnancy test (for HCG, or human chorionic gonadotropin)
- FSH
- LH
- Estradiol (E2)
- TSH (thyroid-stimulating hormone)
- Free T4 (thyroid hormone)
- Prolactin (if elevated, you may have milky breast leakage)
- CBC (complete blood count)
- CMPAN (chemical panel)
- Male hormones (testosterone)
- Pelvic ultrasound

How Is Amenorrhea Treated?

Treatment for amenorrhea depends on the cause and the patient's interests. If you are trying to get pregnant, the first thing is to obtain a pregnancy test. If that is negative, progestin pills, such as Provera (medroxyproges-terone acetate), can be prescribed to bring on a period. The pills are taken for anywhere from 5 to 10 days. Your health care provider may then prescribe a medication by mouth to induce ovulation. The most common ones are clomiphene citrate (Clomid) or letrozole (Femara). These pills are thought to stimulate the pituitary gland to increase output of FSH and LH, thus prompting the ovary to release an egg. There are different doses prescribed depending on the response of the ovary. If a low dose does not work, then a higher dose is prescribed. Some women do not respond to oral medications and require injections of the actual pituitary gland hormones (FSH and LH) and one to trigger ovulation (HCG). Sometimes in vitro fertilization (IVF) is the best treatment; your doctor will help determine the best course for you.

Lifestyle changes along with diet and exercise programs work well to treat obesity, but patients must "make the decision and stick with the plan." Often a 10% decrease in weight allows the whole ovulation axis to work better.

If you do not want to get pregnant, your health care provider can prescribe a birth control pill to restart your monthly periods and provide the estrogen your body may not be making. Estrogen is important to maintain bones and other parts of the body.

Ebony's Story

I ALWAYS HAD NORMAL PERIODS. They started when I was 12 and came at the exact same time every month. I had cramps, but a Midol or two would take care of them. I was always described as a "happy camper." I was close with my family, especially with my older sister, who was my rock and role model. I graduated from nursing school and worked at our local hospital as a floor nurse. Loved the patients and what I did.

Everything was A-OK until I was 24, and my periods just stopped. I knew I wasn't pregnant, and I wasn't on any birth control. While in the shower one day, I noticed this milky discharge from both my breasts. It only came out when I mashed on them, squeezed the nipple. Then I really got worried when my side vision was not as good as it used to be. Headaches were occurring and I never had them before.

I went to my gynecologist, and she ran a few tests. She said my "prolactin was high" and that I needed to get an MRI of my brain, the pituitary gland specifically. Lo and behold, she had me come back to her office and showed me these films and that I had a pituitary tumor. She called it a macroadenoma. I Googled it and learned it makes prolactin, which is why I had the nipple milky discharge. Then I learned it can grow and affect my vision, and that was why I couldn't see as well on the sides. According to Google, the macroadenoma was affecting my peripheral vision, causing "bitemporal hemianopsia." Wow, what a term! Well, they put me on this medicine called bromocriptine, or Parlodel, to shrink the tumor. It worked! No more breast leakage and my periods came back; my prolactin was now back to normal. Not sure how long I have to be on this medication, but I'm happy again.

• TAKEAWAY POINTS •

The most common cause of no periods (amenorrhea) is pregnancy.

Other conditions causing no periods include:
- polycystic ovaries
- thyroid disease
- prolactin elevation (breast leakage)
- premature ovarian insufficiency (early menopause)

Excessive athletic activity level can cause amenorrhea.

Evaluation involves blood tests and sometimes ultrasound.

Treatment depends on the cause and fertility interest.

• KEY WORDS •

amenorrhea
follicle-stimulating hormone (FSH)
functional hypothalamic amenorrhea (FHA)
gonadotropin-releasing hormone (GnRH)
hypothalamic-pituitary-ovarian axis
luteinizing hormone (LH)

Chapter 8

I Just Can't Stop Bleeding

Abnormal Vaginal Bleeding

I WAS 11 WHEN I STARTED HAVING PERIODS. From the start, my period was like a faucet had been turned on, soaking a pad every hour with clots and bad cramps. After a couple of months of heavy bleeding, scared and confused, I confessed to my mom that something was wrong. This was not what my friends had with their "monthly thing." She agreed and decided that we should see her gynecologist. They ordered a couple of blood tests, and afterward the doctor told me an ultrasound probe would be placed on my tummy. I sighed with relief since I had been worrying myself sick thinking something would be placed in my vagina! My tests showed I had a blood clotting disorder called Von Willebrand disease. This indeed was why my first period and subsequent ones were so heavy. The doctor put me on a birth control pill to prevent further bleeding, and everything was finally under control.

Everything was fine until a number of years later, when my partner and I started trying to have a family. Whoa, the heavy periods from my early teens started again! Again, I visited the gynecologist, who recommended an ultrasound. The results indicated the presence of a fibroid. Given the heavy bleeding, a saline infusion sonogram (also called sonohysterogram) further confirmed fibroids inside my uterus. I knew I wanted to get pregnant, but how could I with "tumors in my uterus"? The doctor talked about an operation, which she called a hysteroscopy. I decided to go with it, and following the surgery six months later, I was actually pregnant. Yeah!!!—*Amala*

What You Need to Know about Heavy Periods

It is common but not normal to have irregular or heavy bleeding with your period. The spectrum of abnormal periods includes bleeding between periods, which is called **metrorrhagia**. Heavy periods are termed **menorrhagia**. Abnormal uterine bleeding is usually due to a lack of ovulation, or anovulation. Not uncommonly, heavy periods result in anemia and require iron therapy.

Let's take a moment to state what is normal for menstrual cycles. According to the American College of Obstetricians and Gynecologists, the average menstrual cycle is 24 to 38 days. Having a period that is less frequent or more frequent is considered "abnormal." The average length of a period is 1 to 8 days. A period that lasts less than 2 days or more than 8 days is considered "abnormal." What is a normal amount of bleeding?

What Causes Heavy Uterine Bleeding?

Heavy menstrual flow can be caused by a variety of factors.

- Problems with ovulation
- Fibroids
- Polyps
- Thyroid disorders
- Sexually transmitted infections
- Blood clotting disorders
- Miscarriage

- Ectopic pregnancy
- Cancer (rarely)

How Will My Doctor Determine the Cause of My Heavy Periods?

Doctors sometimes use the mnemonic PALM-COEIN to determine the possible causes:

P = polyp
A = adenomyosis (endometrial-like tissue grows into wall of uterus)
L = leiomyoma (fibroid)
M = malignancy
C = coagulopathy (abnormal blood clotting)
O = ovulatory dysfunction (irregular periods)
E = endometrial (problem in lining of uterus)
I = iatrogenic (caused by treatment such as chemotherapy)
N = not classified (other causes)

It is a good idea to keep track of your periods by maintaining a "menstrual diary," either on a smartphone app or in a journal. You should note how heavy the flow is; soaking a pad in an hour is considered heavy bleeding. Also write down any pain you have and how bad it is.

How Do You Know If It's Abnormal Vaginal Bleeding?

Your health care provider will start with going over your medical history, followed by physical examination. Lab tests may be ordered, and possibly a pelvic ultrasound.

Lab tests for abnormal vaginal bleeding include:

- Complete blood count (CBC)
- Thyroid function studies (TSH and free T4 screening)
- Pregnancy test (ideally a blood test)
- Coagulation panel if you had heavy bleeding after your first period (menarche)
- Sexually transmitted infections (as indicated)

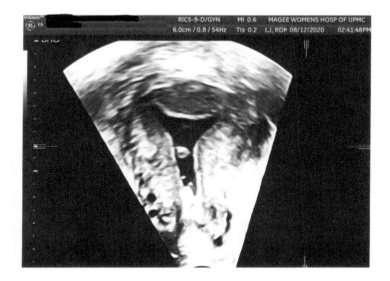

FIGURE 8.1.
Sonohysterogram with polyp.

In some cases, additional imaging will be required to determine the cause of your heavy bleeding. Your doctor may order a pelvic ultrasound (if required) or saline infusion sonogram (sonohysterogram; figure 8.1) if they suspect that you have a fibroid in the lining of uterus.

How Is Heavy Vaginal Bleeding Treated?

Treatment for heavy bleeding depends in part on whether you want to get pregnant. If the answer is, not right now, then there are a number of medical options for treating a heavy period (figure 8.2).

- Birth control pills
- Progestin-only pills
- Nonsteroidal anti-inflammatory drugs, such as ibuprofen
- Tranexamic acid
- Antibiotics for sexually transmitted infections

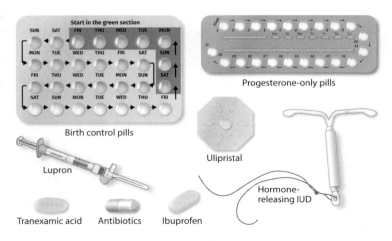

FIGURE 8.2.
Some medical treatment options for abnormal vaginal (uterine) bleeding.

- Hormone-releasing intrauterine devices (Mirena, Kyleena, Skyla, Liletta)
- Medications to shrink fibroids (these stop working once medicine is stopped)
- Gonadotropin-releasing hormone analogues (Lupron, Elagolix)
- Ulipristal (a selective progesterone receptor modulator)

If you are hoping to become pregnant, the treatment for your heavy periods depends on the cause.

- Medications such as Clomid or letrozole to induce ovulation
- Surgery (myomectomy) may be necessary to remove uterine fibroids
- Hysteroscopic myomectomy for fibroids in the uterine lining
- Laparoscopic or open myomectomy for fibroids in other parts of the uterus

If you have completed having children, there are some additional options:

- Endometrial ablation (scars uterine lining)
- Hysterectomy

- Uterine artery embolization (if caused by fibroids)
- Magnetic resonance imaging (MRI)–related procedures
- Focused ultrasound obliteration of the fibroid (also termed HIFU, for high-intensity focused ultrasound ablation of uterine fibroids)

Fatima's Story

I HAD MY FIRST PERIOD when I was 13 years old. I had irregular periods from the beginning. They would come every two weeks and then skip for several months. Over the years I have had a number of problems, like liver abnormalities and anemia. My doctors told me it was due to my smoking.

As I entered my early thirties, I experienced shortness of breath. I have always had a problem with my weight, and headaches with my periods. However, the real big problem was heavy bleeding, with golf-ball-sized clots that would come out of my vagina. On two occasions the bleeding was so bad, I had to go to the emergency room. In fact, I needed a blood transfusion.

I went to my gynecologist after the bleeding, and he examined me and used a term I had never heard before. He said I had a "boggy" uterus. I thought to myself, What is he talking about? He went on to say the uterus was soft, felt "globular," and probably indicated I had a kind of endometriosis in my uterus. I went online and found the word he mentioned, "adenomyosis." The doctor also said he thought there was a fibroid and that I needed to get an ultrasound.

Well, the bleeding occurred several more times, and twice I needed a dilation and curettage (D&C) to control the bleeding. In the meantime, my husband and I decided we wanted to get pregnant. We tried, I guess you would say, since we never used any birth control. I went to my OB-GYN, and he suggested I see an infertility specialist.

That doctor helped me. I had to have the fibroid removed that was in the lining of my uterus. The procedure was called hysteroscopy.

I should mention that I developed a precancer problem in my uterus called "endometrial hyperplasia," which meant I had excessive buildup of the lining of the uterus that needed to be treated with progesterone or progestin for three months before I had the fibroid removed. They said this excessive buildup occurred because of my polycystic ovary syndrome (PCOS), which was diagnosed a while back.

Well, now the bleeding is under control. I feel good, and the infertility doctor said that IVF would give us the best chance of becoming pregnant. We are just embarking on our first IVF cycle; wish us luck!

• TAKEAWAY POINTS •

Abnormal vaginal bleeding requires a pregnancy test.

Thyroid problems can be the cause.

Very heavy bleeding can indicate a blood clotting disorder.

Uterine fibroids are common; treatment depends on their location.

Sexually transmitted infections are occasionally associated with heavy bleeding.

Uterine cancer is rare in women who have menstrual periods but can occur.

• KEY WORDS •

birth control pills
magnetic resonance imaging (MRI)
menorrhagia
metrorrhagia
tranexamic acid

Chapter 9

Painful Periods,
Nobody's Listening

Endometriosis

FOR YEARS, NO DOCTOR TOOK ME SERIOUSLY when I talked about the excruciating pain with my period, which would often leave me bedridden. I just turned 35 last week, and there is not a lot to celebrate since my husband and I have been trying to get pregnant for over a year with no luck so far.

One day, my husband was reading an article on pelvic pain in the local newspaper and turned to me, exclaiming, "Honey, I think you might have endo." I went to my new gynecologist grudgingly but with some sense of hope—this was my sixth gynecologist, after all. She firmly said, "Sabrina, we need to take a look inside. I think this could help your pain and infertility."

I am glad she encouraged me to have laparoscopic surgery, a minimally invasive procedure. Two weeks later, she removed all the endometriosis and suggested that my best chance of pregnancy was over the upcoming year. Her words came true when three months later I was late for my period. However, I wanted to be sure that I was truly pregnant! Sure enough, the doctor confirmed my pregnancy with a blood test, and when

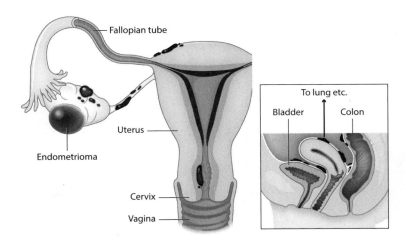

FIGURE 9.1.
Endometriosis involving the ovary (endometrioma) and in locations around the reproductive and other organs.

I heard the heartbeat at six weeks, I cried and cried. It worked. Thank you. Thank you for listening.—*Sabrina*

What You Need to Know about Endometriosis

Endometriosis is a unique medical disease. The uterine lining sheds monthly to produce your period. Endometriosis is defined as a condition where the tissue that is made up of the same cells as the lining of the uterus is present anywhere outside of the uterus. Shedding of this tissue in the abdomen causes irritation, which can lead to **pelvic pain**, scarring, and infertility. Surprisingly, it has been found in unexpected places in the body such as the lungs, the eyes, and in the bowel (figure 9.1).

Do I Have Endometriosis?

You may have endometriosis if you have one or more of the following symptoms.

- Recurrent painful periods
- Inconsistent relief with nonsteroidal medications
- Inconsistent relief with birth control pills
- Painful intercourse, especially with deep penetration
- Premenstrual spotting
- Painful bowel movements during your period
- Family history of endometriosis

The severity of endometriosis does not necessarily match its symptoms. Symptoms can be mild or severe. During your menstrual cycle, the ovarian hormones stimulate the uterine lining. At the same time, the areas of endometriosis outside of the uterus are also stimulated and create symptoms such as painful periods, painful intercourse, and sometimes pain with bowel movements. On the other extreme, a woman with advanced stages of endometriosis may have no symptoms at all.

How Common Is Endometriosis?

Endometriosis affects more than 176 million women worldwide, which is about 10% of women, according to the National Endometriosis Association. Approximately 50% of women who experience repetitive painful periods and difficulty getting pregnant have endometriosis.

What Causes Endometriosis?

Unfortunately, despite all the research on endometriosis, no one knows for sure what causes it. There are some prevailing **theories of endometriosis,** however.

Retrograde menstruation. With each menstrual cycle, every woman has some menstrual flow out of her fallopian tubes and into her abdomen. In some women, when the uterine lining cells deposit on reproductive organs (such as the ovaries), the result is endometriosis.

Circulatory distribution. Endometriosis may be caused when the blood and lymph circulatory systems transport the cells of the uterine lining to several areas in the body.

Coelomic metaplasia. Some women are born with cells in the uterine lining that predispose them to endometriosis. There is some evidence that there may be a genetic component.

Some patients only develop symptoms as they get older.

How Is Endometriosis Diagnosed?

The gold standard in endometriosis diagnosis is **laparoscopy**, which involves surgically looking into the abdomen with a small telescope (laparoscope) and visualizing the reproductive organs. If endometriosis is found, the gynecologic surgeon will address it.

How Does Endometriosis Lead to Infertility?

We do not know exactly why a woman becomes infertile as a result of endometriosis, but two theories may explain the correlation.

1. Endometriosis produces chemicals known as cytokines that disrupt the normal activity of the reproductive organs. In response, the body tries to remove these abnormal areas, creating an immunologic response that can interfere with embryo implantation on the lining of the uterus.
2. Endometriosis has been connected with poor egg quality and scarring, which can cause fallopian tubes to not function properly.

What Is Adenomyosis?

Adenomyosis is a type of endometriosis that has invaded the muscle of the uterus. On physical exam, the uterus feels soft or, in medical terms, "boggy." Similar to endometriosis, symptoms vary; however, the most common symptoms include heavier flow and pain during periods. Unfortunately, there are limited medical treatments for adenomyosis and the best management is a hysterectomy, a surgical procedure to remove the uterus.

How Is Endometriosis Treated?

Treatment for endometriosis depends on the possible cause of the condition, as well as whether you hope to become pregnant. Below are some treatment options.

1. *Birth control pills* inhibit ovulation and sometimes are prescribed continuously to provide more effective pain control.
2. *Nonsteroidals* such as ibuprofen are used as maintenance treatment and can be taken to control pain. This medication can prevent the body from producing prostaglandins, which are chemical substances that cause cramps. Ideally, ibuprofen would be started one to two days prior to periods.
3. *Other medications* such as leuprolide can be used to create a temporary medical menopause. A few trade names for leuprolide are Lupron, Elagolix, Eligard, Viadur, and Leupromer. Aromatase inhibitors such as letrozole can be used to treat endometriosis by inhibiting estrogen production. Following treatment, you can try to get pregnant.
4. Overall, one of the best treatments for endometriosis is *pregnancy* because the reproductive hormones provide a beneficial effect.

Your health care professional may suggest proceeding with in vitro fertilization (IVF). In general, depending on the stage, patient age, and other factors, the presence of endometriosis does not seem to affect the success of IVF.

Maggie's Story

FROM THE OUTSIDE LOOKING IN, I had a normal high school experience. I played on a sports team, had a great group of friends, and did well in my classes. But in private, I struggled with the most debilitating periods. They would be irregular and sometimes heavy at the beginning, but the most unbearable part was the pain—my back, my stomach—it was so bad it would make me double over. Advil or Tylenol would offer relief only for a few hours, and I found myself missing school often. Desperate and in pain, I wound up seeing four different doctors and was left asking myself, What now?

Finally, I dragged myself to a fifth doctor. Walking into the waiting room with Mom and Dad, I saw a couple of other young women like me. The good vibes from the lobby translated to a meaningful conversation with my doctor. He said, "You are 17, have not had relief with any medication or lifestyle change so far, and I'm sorry that you continue to experience this pain."

"Looks like endometriosis," he said after he did an ultrasound and found a cyst on my ovary. We discussed two options: medical treatment or surgery to remove the endometriosis that was causing me pain. I wanted it removed, so surgery it was. The surgery itself took four hours, and apparently the doctor found endometriosis everywhere; it was on my bowel, my ovaries, and around my rectum—which explains my painful poops! The doctor got it all out, and I was pain-free for years.

I am 27 now, and my husband and I have been trying to get pregnant for a frustrating amount of time. I am starting to have pain with sex, so we have tried changing positions, which would sometimes stop the pain. However, now it's so excruciating that we have to stop. My cramps are back, and I'm realizing that I had never considered if my earlier endometriosis could affect pregnancy. I went to a reproductive endocrinologist—an OB-GYN that specializes in infertility—and shared my frustration with him. He was understanding, just like the previous doctor who operated on me. We discussed my options to pursue pregnancy, but all I could think about was my pain.

I had brought my medical records from the first surgery, and my doctor quickly pointed to a finding on the operative report: endometriosis. He shared with me that a similar operation would be recommended to relieve the pain, but also might help the sperm and egg meet so I could get pregnant. The latter would be facilitated by removing "adhesions," or scarring around my tubes. He wanted me to be seen by a gynecologic surgeon who specializes in this type of surgery.

He referred me to a minimally invasive gynecologic surgeon (MIGS). She said I was "full of endometriosis" but that she was able to remove it from my tubes and ovaries during the operation. She advised that we would have our best chance to get pregnant this upcoming year.

I knew right away something good had been done because there was no pain with sex, no pain with periods, and no pain with bowel movements. I let myself get excited and would check my ovulation app constantly. Midcycle, I would repeatedly say, "Today's the day, honey."

It is now six months later, and my reproductive endocrinologist just confirmed a healthy pregnancy in my uterus by ultrasound. It matched with my delayed period and pregnancy test, but I needed this confirmation for so many reasons!

• TAKEAWAY POINTS •

Pelvic pain *is real* and should not be ignored. Seek help from your health care professional if you have pain with sex, periods, or bowel movements.

Endometriosis is essentially when the cells lining the uterine cavity grow outside the uterus.

Treatment for endometriosis is unique to your fertility goals.

Endometriosis requires a surgical diagnosis.

The best time to attempt pregnancy for women suffering from endometriosis is immediately following surgery to remove the endometrial tissue.

IVF success in general, depending upon stage, may not be affected by the extent of endometriosis.

• KEY WORDS •

adenomyosis
endometriosis
family history
laparoscopy
pelvic pain
theories of endometriosis

Chapter 10

I Have Acne, I'm Hairy, and I Just Can't Get Pregnant

Polycystic Ovaries

I AM 24 YEARS OLD and have struggled with acne since I was a teenager. I have hair seemingly everywhere—it's constantly growing on my chin and upper lip, and I have to shave at least once a week. It's so embarrassing! I've struggled with my weight for most of my life. I exercise like crazy, and you name the diet, I have tried it. But I just can't seem to keep the weight off. Bob and I got married a while ago, and we have been trying to get pregnant for over a year. My periods are irregular, so I am never sure whether I'm ovulating. You name the ovulation predictor kit, I have bought it. Oddly, every time I check it, it's positive. I'm getting more and more depressed as time goes on, losing hope. What do I do, and who do I turn to?—*Monica*

What You Need to Know about Polycystic Ovarian Syndrome

The most common hormonal problem among women is polycystic ovaries, or better termed **polycystic ovarian syndrome (PCOS)**. Overall, 10% of women have PCOS. Typically, the condition is associated with **acne**, hair growth (**hirsutism**), and **irregular periods**. One of the underlying problems is increased insulin levels (hyperinsulinemia), which is associated with increased pigmentation of the skin on the back of the neck and underarms. This darkening of the skin is called acanthosis. Other possible complications include developing **diabetes** during pregnancy (gestational diabetes), high blood pressure, anxiety, depression, thinning of the hair, and sleep apnea. Patients, long term, are prone to developing diabetes (type 2) and sometimes early heart attacks. Often there is a family history of PCOS and women in the family developing adult-onset diabetes (type 2). One other concern is having long intervals between periods. In this situation, the lining of the uterus tends to build up more than normal, a condition called endometrial hyperplasia, which can occasionally lead to cancer of the uterus.

What Are the Symptoms of Polycystic Ovarian Syndrome?

Some of the symptoms of PCOS include the following (figure 10.1).

- Acne
- Hair growth (hirsutism)
- Irregular periods
- Weight gain

What Tests Will I Need?

Your primary health care provider may order a test of one or more of the following to help make a diagnosis of PCOS. These tests are important, as they can help rule in or out other conditions that may be contributing to your symptoms.

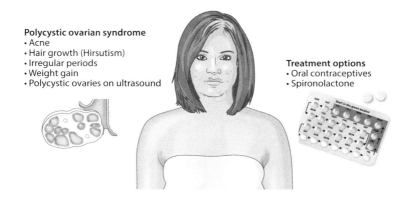

Polycystic ovarian syndrome
- Acne
- Hair growth (Hirsutism)
- Irregular periods
- Weight gain
- Polycystic ovaries on ultrasound

Treatment options
- Oral contraceptives
- Spironolactone

FIGURE 10.1.
Diagnosis and treatment of polycystic ovarian syndrome.

- Testosterone
- DHEA-S: a male hormone from the adrenal gland
- 17- hydroxyprogesterone: to distinguish PCOS from other problems, such as adult-onset congenital adrenal hyperplasia (a genetic disorder that affects the adrenal glands)
- Hemoglobin A1c (HgbA1c): average blood sugar level
- Pelvic ultrasound to look for polycystic ovaries

How Does a Health Care Provider Make the Diagnosis?

A diagnosis of PCOS is primarily made by the patient's history, including:

- Irregular periods
- Evidence of increased male hormones (androgens)
- Polycystic-appearing ovaries on ultrasound (figure 10.2)

If you have two of three of the above symptoms and your doctor has eliminated other problems related to the adrenal gland, you will receive a diagnosis of PCOS. These criteria are called the **Rotterdam criteria** for polycystic ovaries.

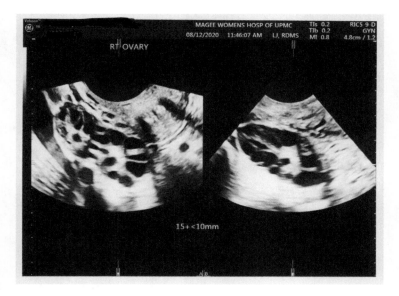

FIGURE 10.2.
Polycystic ovaries on ultrasound.

Can PCOS Be Treated?

The best treatment for PCOS is often a change in lifestyle, which means diet and exercise. Eating healthy and exercising regularly are key, but any behavioral change has to be something that you can reasonably fit into your daily routine. Success in this area can lead to more regular periods, pregnancy, and lower chances of developing diabetes and heart-related problems.

What If You Have PCOS and Want to Get Pregnant?

If you want to get pregnant and have especially irregular periods, your doctor may prescribe pills to help you ovulate. The most common treatments are **Clomid** (clomiphene citrate) and **letrozole** (Femara). These pills are usually started after a period and taken for 5 days per month, with the expectation that ovulation will take place around 10 days after taking the pills. Unfortunately, ovulation predictor kits do not always work well because the hormone they detect, LH (luteinizing hormone), which normally increases right before ovulation, is already at a high level in women with PCOS.

You may be a candidate for in vitro fertilization if the ovulation-inducing medications do not work. Most women with PCOS who get pregnant do well and have a baby. They do have a higher chance of miscarriage, however, and some studies have found that women with PCOS have a greater chance of developing high blood pressure during pregnancy. In addition, women with PCOS may develop gestational diabetes mellitus.

Does Treatment Differ If Pregnancy Is Not Desired?

If you don't want to get pregnant, birth control pills, progestin-only pills (POPs), and spironolactone (which helps with acne and excessive hair growth) are options. We often place a patient who does not want to get pregnant on birth control pills to both prevent excessive buildup of the uterine lining, termed endometrial protection, and to control acne and hair growth (hirsutism). Birth control pills have several other advantages, such as lowering a woman's chance of developing cancer of the ovaries, uterus, and to some extent the colon. A disadvantage, though rare, includes the chance of developing a blood clot, usually in the legs.

Are There Other Treatments for PCOS?

You may have heard of metformin, which is a medication that helps to better utilize insulin in your body. It is approved by the US Food and Drug Administration to treat type 2 diabetes but has been shown to aid in weight reduction for people with PCOS. Metformin can also help lower cholesterol. As far as helping you to get pregnant, recent studies have not found that metformin helps to stimulate ovulation. Metformin may have side effects, including nausea and diarrhea.

In large part, your treatment will depend on what your immediate plans are. If you are not planning pregnancy, then ovulation prevention medications (birth control pills are a good choice) should be considered. It is a good idea to keep track of your periods (either with a journal or a smartphone app; see chapter 2).

Spironolactone (Aldactone) can be prescribed to treat acne and excessive hair growth, but you must not get pregnant on this medication (use effective birth control). Taking spironolactone during pregnancy can cause birth defects of the genitalia.

If you are planning pregnancy, ovulation-inducing medicines such as Clomid or letrozole, taken by mouth, will often result in ovulation. Timing of intercourse is key as the next step. Side effects of these ovulation-inducing medications include hot flashes, dryness with intercourse, and rarely multiple fetuses. If there is one most important recommendation, it is to make changes to your lifestyle. Weight reduction along with a healthy diet and exercise program tend to allow better utilization of insulin and may well allow ovulation to occur or the medications to work more effectively. In vitro fertilization remains an option when other treatments don't work.

Genevieve's Story

AS A TEENAGER, I was always concerned about acne. I saw a dermatologist who prescribed a bunch of medications to apply to my face. I was placed on Accutane and had to sign a paper that I would use birth control if sexually active. Well, the good news is it worked and improved my skin. As I entered my early twenties, I began to grow hair on my face. It was so bad I had to shave every other day—how embarrassing! I was never the most popular girl, but I did have dates and hung out with friends in college and stuff. Well, soon after I graduated, the man of my dreams walked into my life. We got married and thought we would live happily ever after or something like that. We began to focus on getting pregnant. We did not use any birth control, but my periods were very irregular. Time marched on and nothing, I mean nothing! Those dumb old ovulation predictor kits never worked! They would always come up positive.

I mustered up the courage to go to my doctor, who said we should try some Clomid. I took a pill a day for five days and got a period but no pregnancy. We did that three times, after which my doctor said I should see a specialist. I went to his office and met the PA (physician assistant), who was great and very informative. She recommended we have an evaluation to see what the problem was. I had blood tests and an ultrasound, and my husband had a semen analysis. When we went back to go over the results, I was a nervous wreck. The PA was very nice and explained that the tests indicated I have polycystic ovaries. She said the irregular periods, the acne, hair growth (she used the word "hirsutism"), and the ultrasound of my ovaries all pointed to PCOS, or polycystic ovarian syndrome. She said it's common, and that 10% of women have it.

We talked about treatment, and she said since I was on Clomid with no success, we should try something called letrozole. She said it is taken by mouth for five days and that I should have sex when I think I might be ovulating. Wow, after the first cycle, I was late for my period and went and got a home pregnancy test. I peed on the stick and voila—it was POSITIVE. I screamed in the bathroom! In tears, I immediately called my husband. He said I better check back with the doctor's office. I called, and they had me come in for a blood pregnancy test. It was positive and a good number, but they wanted me to recheck the blood test in two days to see if it doubled. Yes indeed! Then they said you need an ultrasound at around six weeks. At that appointment I heard it—a tiny little heartbeat. Let's fast-forward to our daughter—she's incredible, and we love her to death. We are happy campers, have our precious little girl, a dog named Molly, and I have a great husband. Now we are thinking about a second baby. I hope the doctor or PA will give me that letrozole again.

• **TAKEAWAY POINTS** •

For patients with PCOS, lifestyle (diet and exercise) is key.

Treatment for ovulation may be required (Clomid or letrozole).

Acne and hirsutism can be treated medically, but the treatment will depend on whether a pregnancy is desired.

If you are not planning a pregnancy, birth control pills can alleviate the symptoms of PCOS.

• **KEY WORDS** •

acne
Clomid
diabetes
hirsutism
irregular periods
letrozole
polycystic ovarian syndrome (PCOS)
weight gain

_____

Chapter 11

No Room for the Fetus

Uterine Fibroids

MY MENSTRUAL FLOW HAS INCREASED; I soak a tampon in about an hour. If I have to get up in the middle of the night to urinate, not a lot of urine comes out. I am a teacher and recently noted that I have to excuse myself from my class to pee, and again not a lot comes out. I'm frustrated! My husband, Shawn, and I are trying to get pregnant, and we time sex with an ovulation predictor app month after month. I went to the doctor, and she told me, "I think you have fibroids." She said they were large when she examined me with a pelvic exam. She went on to say they are probably compressing my bladder and that's why small amounts of urine come out and I have to go more often. I asked what about my heavy periods; she said the fibroids are probably in the lining of my uterus. Now what? She said we are going to do tests that will include an ultrasound of my pelvis. I hope they can treat me with medicine and I won't have to have surgery.—*Liya*

What You Need to Know about Uterine Fibroids

Uterine **fibroids**, also termed leiomyoma, are not cancerous. They are benign, smooth-muscle tumors of the uterus. The most common gynecologic problem among women of reproductive age (18 to 49 years), fibroids usually do not have any symptoms; however, just as in Liya's case, they can cause **heavy vaginal bleeding**, pelvic pressure, bladder compression, and infertility. There appears to be a genetic component, and studies have shown that race may play a role. African American women have a higher chance of developing fibroids. Fibroids usually get smaller after menopause. In women of reproductive age, up to 49 years old, fibroids can change the shape of the inside of the uterus, meaning the uterine lining, causing embryo implantation problems and thus infertility. If you get pregnant, fibroids can affect how the pregnancy progresses. About 10% to 30% of patients with fibroids have associated pregnancy complications and problems at delivery.

Fibroids and Pregnancy Complications

Even though fibroids are benign, they can cause complications during pregnancy, including:

- Miscarriage
- Bleeding in early pregnancy
- Preterm labor
- Preterm delivery
- Abnormal fetal presentation
- Postpartum bleeding
- Retained placenta
- Intrauterine growth restriction
- Placental abruption
- Rarely, uterine rupture after removal of fibroids (myomectomy)

The size and location of the fibroid or fibroids can affect your ability to get pregnant. Health care professionals use the following terms to describe the location of fibroids.

Submucosal: in the cavity of the uterus
Intramural: in the muscle of the uterus

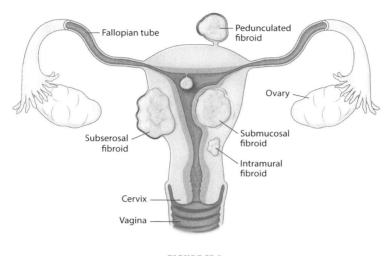

FIGURE 11.1.
Types of uterine fibroids.

Subserosal: toward the outside of the uterus

Pedunculated: attached but hanging off the uterus

A diagram of the female reproductive anatomy that shows where fibroids may be located in and around the uterus is shown in figure 11.1.

Submucosal fibroids, which sit right in the inner lining of the uterus, are the most concerning type for fertility purposes because they interfere with implantation of the embryo. Submucosal fibroids cause a change in the shape of the inner uterine cavity and can prevent an embryo from implanting.

Size and location are key factors, and while there is no specific cutoff, in general when a fibroid is larger than 4–5 centimeters (about 2 inches in diameter), it can interfere with fertility. Subserosal fibroids (those located toward the outside of the uterus) do not tend to have as bad an effect on pregnancy and fertility in general.

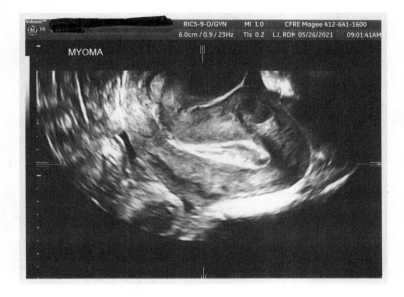

FIGURE 11.2.
Ultrasound of fibroids.

What Are the Signs and Symptoms of Fibroids?

- Heavy uterine bleeding
- Pelvic pain and pressure
- Infertility
- Miscarriage
- Pelvic pain during pregnancy, when fibroids outgrow their blood supply (known as degeneration)
- Growth of fibroids from pregnancy hormones
- Interference with labor and delivery

Diagnosis of fibroids is based on your symptoms and a physical examination (especially the pelvic exam and imaging of your uterus). The most common way to look at the uterus is through **ultrasound** with a vaginal probe (figure 11.2). If the doctor needs more information regarding the location of the fibroids, a **sonohysterogram** (also known as a saline infusion sonogram) can be done. Here, a tiny tube is placed into the vagina, through the cervix, and into the cavity of the uterus. Then, saline is flushed in the cavity of the uterus. We watch the saline fill the cavity of the uterus with ultrasound in real time to see if there is any area that disturbs the cavity. Normally, the cavity looks like a black triangle with smooth walls, but if you have submucosal fibroids, they appear as bumps within the triangle. Sometimes the fallopian tubes are also checked at the time of sonohysterogram. Such imaging requires a small amount of air and saline, and looking on an ultrasound for fluid coming out of the tubes. Other imaging includes **magnetic resonance imaging (MRI)** and rarely computed tomography (CT) to evaluate fibroids.

Treatment depends on your symptoms and fertility interests. Medical treatment only appears to shrink the fibroid while you are taking it. As soon as the treatment is stopped, the fibroids go back to their original size.

What Are the Medical Treatments for Fibroids?

There are several medications that are prescribed to treat fibroids. Below are brand-name medications; generic formulations may also be available.

1. Gonadotropin-releasing agonists: Lupron, Elagolix, Zoladex, Trelstar
2. Levonorgesterol-releasing intrauterine devices: Mirena, Liletta, Skyla
3. Nonsteroidal anti-inflammatory drugs (NSAIDs): Motrin, Advil
4. Progestin-only oral contraceptives: Camilla
5. Estrogen- and progestin-containing oral contraceptives: Loestrin
6. Selective progesterone receptor modulators: Mifeprex
7. Selective estrogen receptor modulators: Evista, Nolvadex
8. Tranexamic acid: Lysteda
9. Ulipristal: Ella
10. Aromatase inhibitors: Armidex, Femara

In a patient who desires pregnancy and decides to treat the fibroids surgically, the type of surgery will depend on fibroid location. A submucosal fibroid (or one that is in the uterine cavity) is usually treated with hysteroscopic myomectomy. In this procedure, an instrument called a hysteroscopic resectoscope is passed through the vagina and cervix and into the uterus. Then the portion of the fibroid that is in the uterus is shaved down. This seems to work well and probably allows the uterine lining to grow in a more normal manner. Sometimes the entire fibroid can be removed via hysteroscopy. If there are fibroids in the uterine muscle (intramural) or toward the outside (subserosal), your options to hysteroscopic myomectomy are a laparoscopic myomectomy, which is done through small incisions in the abdomen, or an open surgical procedure, laparotomy, to remove the fibroids. After a laparoscopy or laparotomy, the patient almost always needs a cesarean section when giving birth, as the uterus in rare occasions may rupture during labor.

If pregnancy is not desired, other approaches to treatment of fibroids, such as endometrial ablation (where a thin layer of tissue, the lining of the uterine cavity [endometrium], is removed) and myolysis (focused energy destruction of the fibroid), can be considered. These procedures are not advised if you want to become pregnant, as they can compromise chances of carrying a baby. Sometimes, if a woman has completed her childbearing and does not want a hysterectomy, **uterine artery embolization (UAE)** can be done to shrink the fibroids by cutting off their blood supply, but here too subsequent pregnancy is not advised.

Ainsley's Story

I AM 16 AND EXPERIENCING PELVIC PRESSURE and having to pee frequently. Something is wrong, I thought to myself. I told my mom about it, and she took me to our doctor, who referred me to an oncologist and surgeon. They were concerned that I had a rapidly growing tumor in my abdomen. I was scared, like really scared! I might mention I was having heavy vaginal bleeding, like I never had before. They talked to me and my parents and said they needed to get a diagnosis. The suggestion was "laparoscopy"—I think I am saying that correctly. They would get a biopsy of the tumor using a telescope that would be placed at my belly button. I Googled it and learned that when the uterus grows fast like this, what they were thinking, it could be a cancer called a "sarcoma." OMG, what do we do now? I had no other choice than to go with the surgery.

Thank heavens it was benign; the doctors said it was a large fibroid. The task of treating it then began. The doctors threw out all kinds of drug names—I remember Lupron, I think there was something called ulipristal (never heard of it before), and birth control pills. I met all kinds of specialists. There was a pediatric gynecologist, a reproductive endocrinologist, another oncologist. All I seemed to do was see doctors all day long. I am in high school; this shouldn't be my life. I am an athlete and very good student. All this stuff was getting in the way!

I even had a radiologist (I think he said he was an "interventional radiologist") say they could put a tube, a "catheter," in my groin to access the uterus blood supply and block it to shrink the uterus tumors, but this procedure could affect my ability to have a baby. I didn't like that option; I want to have kids someday. Well, I wound up with an operation called myomectomy. Boy, was I scared. The doctors told me it was possible I could end up having a hysterectomy. I have a scar on my belly that is pretty big. Thankfully, the surgery went well, and they took out all the fibroids. Then they put me on medicine, Lupron, to shrink any new fibroids. I've been doing well so far. I still have my uterus and hope to have babies one day.

• TAKEAWAY POINTS •

Fibroids are common.

The fibroid location and size are important factors in treatment.

Most patients with fibroids do not have problems with pregnancy.

The miscarriage rate is somewhat higher among women who have fibroids.

Pain during pregnancy is usually due to the changes fibroids are undergoing (degeneration).

Non-hysteroscopic myomectomy usually means that a cesarean section during childbirth will be necessary.

Endometrial ablation, myolysis, and uterine artery embolization are not good treatment options if you want to get pregnant.

Surgery depends on the fibroid's location and may improve your chances of a successful pregnancy.

• KEY WORDS •

fibroid
heavy vaginal bleeding
magnetic resonance imaging (MRI)
sonohysterogram
submucosal, intramural, subserosal, and pedunculated fibroids
ultrasound
uterine artery embolization (UAE)

Chapter 12

Too Little, Too Early

Miscarriages

I'M SOBBING BECAUSE it's happening again. I'm late for my period. I just did a home pregnancy test, and it's positive. I call my doctor, and she says to come in for a blood pregnancy test. I would ordinarily be very excited, but this is the third time this has happened. Twice I went as far as to have an ultrasound. The first one showed a pregnancy in the uterus, and the second one a heartbeat. Once again I was thrilled beyond belief, but only a week later I started noticing some bleeding. I called my doctor, who said I should come in so I could get an ultrasound. The baby died—she called it an "embryonic demise." Then we had to go through the choices, whether we wanted to wait and see if I passed the pregnancy. I thought, My Lord, I can't do this. There was discussion about what she called "medical treatment," which included taking pills to help the pregnancy pass. Then she said we could manage the pregnancy surgically by doing a procedure called a dilation and curettage (D&C) to get the tissue out of the uterus and send some of it for genetic testing. I had to call my husband because it was all just so frightening. Why does this have to happen to me?—*Samantha*

What You Need to Know about Miscarriage

Also called **spontaneous abortion**, a **miscarriage** is the loss of a pregnancy before the 20th week. If you have had a miscarriage, know that you are not alone. Some 10% to 20% of all pregnancies result in a miscarriage. We know that if a woman is over 40 years of age, the chance of miscarriage goes up to 40%. The total number of miscarriages is probably higher if you include a late period with a positive blood pregnancy test (BHCG hormone)—what we call a **chemical pregnancy**; this increases the number to 30% to 40% of all pregnancies. But we don't really count chemical pregnancies in terms of total number of pregnancies. Even with all of these statistics, at the end of the day, we often don't know why many miscarriages occur.

There are many factors that contribute to becoming pregnant, and even someone who does everything right can have a miscarriage. If you or someone you know has had a miscarriage, you know the emotional toll it takes. Everyone processes grief differently, and there is no "right" way to process loss. Many understandably report anger, anxiety, sadness, and depression.

If you find that your grief symptoms are lasting longer and starting to affect the things that you normally enjoy, reach out to anyone you can share these feelings with, whether it be a family member, friend, or coworker. Know more than anything that a miscarriage is not your fault. If you feel you need psychological support, reach out to your doctor or health care provider.

What Are the Signs and Symptoms of Miscarriage?

Call your health care provider if you experience any of the following during early pregnancy.

- Vaginal bleeding
- Cramps
- Passage of clots or clumps of tissue

What Are the Risk Factors for Miscarriage?

Certain conditions and risk factors may make a miscarriage more likely.

- Advanced maternal age (over 35 years old)
- Smoking
- Obesity
- Diabetes
- Thyroid disease
- Drug and alcohol use
- Very rarely, amniocentesis

Overall, most miscarriages occur during the **first trimester** (the first 13 weeks) and usually are due to a genetic problem with the embryo. Genetic defects are often recognized in cross-talk between the uterine lining and the embryo, which are key factors in implantation. The abnormal genetics of the embryo can result in a "blighted ovum" or "embryonic demise." Most of the time the uterus expels the abnormal pregnancy, but sometimes medication or a **dilation and curettage** (**D&C**) to remove the pregnancy tissue is required. In some cases, not all of the pregnancy is expelled during miscarriage. This is termed incomplete abortion, and here again a D&C may be required. It is important to ask your health care provider if you have an Rh-negative blood type that you get an injection of Rhogam right after the miscarriage or with bleeding during pregnancy, as this will minimize future pregnancy-related problems with the fetus's blood cells.

Chromosomal abnormalities are more common in women over 40 years old. The most common chromosomal abnormalities with miscarriage are:

- Aneuploidy: abnormal chromosome number or defect in one or more chromosomes
- Autosomal trisomy: three copies of one gene

- Monosomy X: missing one X or Y chromosome
- Triploidy: tripling of the chromosome number

Second- and third-trimester miscarriages take on a whole new series of causes. Second-trimester miscarriages (those that occur at 13–26 weeks) are more often due to an abnormality involving the anatomy of the uterus, such as a septum (where a membrane divides the inside of the uterus) or abnormal shape, or bicornuate (or two separate) uteruses and cervixes (what is termed as a didelphic uterus). Fibroids can cause miscarriage, as can a cervix that dilated too soon (known as an incompetent cervix). Infection such as chorioamnionitis, especially in the third trimester (27–40 weeks), and problems with the placenta, like separating off (placental abruption), can result in preterm delivery of the baby. Surgery (such as to remove the appendix or gall bladder) as well as urinary tract infections can also cause miscarriage and early delivery.

If you have had more than two miscarriages, you have what doctors call recurrent pregnancy loss, which may warrant evaluation to determine the cause.

What Causes Recurrent Miscarriages?

Genetic (chromosomal) abnormalities of the mother or father can result in an embryo that is genetically abnormal. Balanced translocation occurs when chromosomes attach to the wrong place when forming the new embryo. This condition can lead to recurrent miscarriages.

Anatomic conditions such as uterine abnormality and hormonal conditions such as thyroid disease, diabetes, and inadequate progesterone from the ovary also contribute to pregnancy loss. As discussed in chapter 5, an immunologic response may be to blame for rejection of pregnancy soon after implantation.

As depicted in figure 12.1, miscarriages can be "threatened," meaning the patient has bleeding but there is evidence that the pregnancy is in the uterus and viable. "Inevitable" means the cervix is open and a mis-

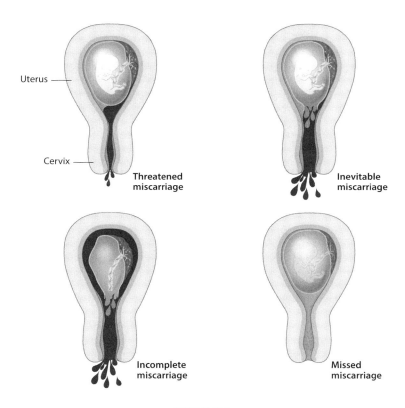

Uterus

Cervix

Threatened
miscarriage

Inevitable
miscarriage

Incomplete
miscarriage

Missed
miscarriage

FIGURE 12.1.
The types of miscarriage.

carriage is imminent. "Incomplete" means some of the pregnancy tissue has been passed and some remains in the uterus. "Missed" means the pregnancy/embryo or fetus has died and remains in the uterus.

Scarring in the uterus can occur following a miscarriage or a term pregnancy when there is a need for a D&C. We do not understand why some women and not others develop this condition, commonly known as Asherman syndrome after the doctor who first reported it. It usually is associated with absence of periods or significant decrease in menstrual flow. Treatment of Asherman syndrome is hysteroscopy with removal of the scarring (hysteroscopic lysis of adhesions). This is usually followed by hormonal treatment, and many times a device such as a balloon or catheter is placed in the uterus for 7 to 14 days. All of these measures are to minimize recurrence of scarring.

Maintaining good prenatal care; following a healthy lifestyle; avoiding smoking, drugs, and alcohol; and addressing medical problems before you get pregnant is wise advice. You should also take prenatal vitamins, which include folic acid, to aid in fetal development and as part of good nutrition for you and your baby.

Alissia's Story

MY STORY BEGINS WITH HAVING five miscarriages. Every one of them began with my pregnancy blood test being positive. I went 16 weeks and then went into what they called "premature labor," and that was the end of the pregnancy. Then I had one where they said the pregnancy was in the uterus, but it didn't progress. My last pregnancy I started bleeding heavily, like soaking a pad in no time. I went to the emergency room, and the doctor said he needed to page "the OB on call" since I didn't have my own doctor and needed a D&C. I went to the operating room shaking, sobbing, and feeling out of control. Everyone was great; the anesthetist made me feel at ease. She gave me medicine through my IV, and I relaxed. Next thing I remember is waking up in the recovery room. I went home and didn't have a period for months. I knew something bad occurred. I went to a fertility specialist, and he did an ultrasound with water, I think it was saline, inside my uterus and said I had extensive scarring, probably from the miscarriage D&C. He said he could operate and fix the problem. I went back to surgery and when I came out, he said I had a balloon in my uterus, would need to be on antibiotics for a short time while I had the balloon in, and needed to take estrogen to help heal the lining of my uterus. The balloon came out 10 days later, and couple of weeks after that I had a period. Thank God! The doctor did another of those ultrasounds and said the lining looked good. We tried on our own, and on the third cycle, I was pregnant. The doctor said my uterus looked good, and the baby had a heartbeat. Well, now I'm 20 weeks and so far, so good. But they did tell me I might have a problem with the placenta growing into the wall of the uterus. Keep your fingers crossed for me!

• TAKEAWAY POINTS •

Approximately 10% of pregnancies result in miscarriages.

Most miscarriages are due to embryo genetic abnormalities that are not at all related to the mother.

Vaginal bleeding, cramps, and sometimes tissue passage occur during a miscarriage.

Recurrent miscarriage is defined as having three or more miscarriages, but evaluation can be done after two miscarriages.

Evaluation specifics depend on what trimester the miscarriages take place in.

It is best to address risk factors before getting pregnant, if possible.

Asherman syndrome is scarring in the cavity of the uterus.

• KEY WORDS •

chemical pregnancy
chromosomal abnormalities
dilation and curettage (D&C)
first trimester
miscarriage
recurrent pregnancy loss
spontaneous abortion
vaginal bleeding

Chapter 13

Wrong Place, Painful Conception

Ectopic Pregnancy

FIRST TIME I EVER HAD SEX was as a senior in high school. I was always attentive in health class and learned about sexually transmitted diseases and how they could affect your future ability to get pregnant. I made a decision that going on birth control pills was all I needed to feel safe having sex. Later on in my life, when I was 30 years old, I got married and decided I would like to have a baby, so I stopped taking birth control pills and tried to get pregnant. Three months later, I was late for my period. This was very unusual, as my periods were like clock-work every 30 days since I stopped the pills. I rushed out to get a home pregnancy test and indeed it was positive. Elated, I thought it was time to celebrate, but then I noticed a little spotting and experienced pain in my lower right abdomen. Oh dear, I thought, could it be my appendix? I went to my doctor, who examined me and did a blood pregnancy test (quantitative human chorionic gonadotropin, or HCG). The doctor and team told me to get a second pregnancy test in two days. The physician assistant then called and said that my pregnancy test was not doubling every two days as in a normal pregnancy. She suggested an ultrasound. No pregnancy was in the uterus nor in a fallopian tube. They told me it was a "pregnancy of unknown location," or PUL. I was worried but still hopeful. Bad turned to worse, and my pain got so severe that I wound up in the emergency room. The doctors did a pregnancy test, which was positive, and a bedside ultrasound of my uterus and tubes. They told me blood was in my belly, a lot of it. Then my blood pressure was going down, and I could feel my heart racing. I remember hearing the word "shock." Next thing I know, I was whisked off to the operating room. When the doctors conducted a laparoscopy (where they put a telescope in my belly), they found a ruptured ectopic pregnancy. Unfortunately, my damaged fallopian tube had to be removed. Thankfully, I did well following surgery.—*Daphne*

What You Need to Know about Ectopic Pregnancy

Ectopic pregnancy is a pregnancy located outside the uterus. It is usually in the fallopian tube but can occur on an ovary, in a C-section scar, in the cervix, or in the abdomen (figure 13.1).

The classic signs of an ectopic pregnancy include:

- Late period
- Vaginal bleeding
- Abdominal pain (sharp, dull, or crampy)

Women who have a history of **sexually transmitted infection** such as chlamydia or gonorrhea have an increased risk of ectopic pregnancy. Chlamydia in particular is what we call a "silent epidemic." It can produce damage to the fallopian tube, setting the stage for an ectopic pregnancy

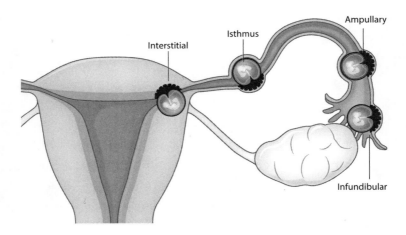

FIGURE 13.1.
Most common locations for tubal ectopic pregnancy.

while the patient does not even know she has it. In part, this is why we do sexually transmitted infection screening in sexually active women, especially if they have more than one partner.

What Are the Causes of Ectopic Pregnancy?

In addition to sexually transmitted infections like chlamydia, there are several risk factors that make an ectopic pregnancy more likely:

- Pelvic inflammatory disease (PID)
- Smoking
- Tubal surgery
- Endometriosis
- Prior ectopic pregnancy
- Becoming pregnant after a tubal ligation
- Becoming pregnant while using an intrauterine device (IUD)
- Being over 35 years of age
- In vitro fertilization (rarely)

When health care providers assess a pregnancy, they use a quantitative blood pregnancy test to check that **human chorionic gonadotropin (HCG)**, a hormone produced early on in the pregnancy, is doubling (or at least increasing 35%) every 48 hours. An ultrasound usually reveals a sac in the uterus at five to six weeks of pregnancy at the same time the blood pregnancy test (serum HCG) is around 1,500 to 2,500 mIU/ml. We call this the "discriminatory zone." Your health care professional may measure your blood progesterone level, which is sometimes used with serum HCG as an indicator of ectopic pregnancy. If your progesterone level is below 10 ng/ml, it indicates an abnormal pregnancy. Ectopic pregnancies often appear as an enlargement of the fallopian tube on transvaginal ultrasound. A ruptured ectopic can be a life-threatening emergency. Overall, the rate of ectopic pregnancy is 1% to 2% of all pregnancies. Unfortunately, up to 10% of women may have no signs or symptoms.

Why Does an Ectopic Pregnancy Occur?

Ectopic pregnancy can occur if the woman has a prior sexually transmitted infection that has damaged the lining (the cilia) of the fallopian tube. In this case, the egg, which is normally fertilized in the tube, begins to grow and becomes stuck journeying toward the uterus. Prior abdominal surgery can cause adhesions or scar tissue around the tube and alter tubal activity, also setting the stage for an ectopic pregnancy. There is also the rare situation where two simultaneous pregnancies occur in the uterus and in the fallopian tube. This is termed "heterotopic pregnancy."

How Is an Ectopic Pregnancy Treated?

Treatment of ectopic pregnancy depends on a number of factors, including how far along the pregnancy is, the blood pregnancy (HCG) value, the picture on a pelvic ultrasound that may or may not include cardiac activity of the embryo, and the patient's symptoms. Occasionally, an ectopic is just monitored with blood pregnancy tests. We call this wait-and-see approach "expectant management." Your health care provider will discuss options with you as indicated.

Medical treatment may involve having **methotrexate** administered as an injection. It requires a blood test to check liver function and an ultrasound. Ideally, the size of the ectopic is 3.5 centimeters or smaller and there is no cardiac activity on ultrasound. If your doctor determines that you have an ectopic pregnancy, you will be asked to stop taking all prenatal vitamins and other folic acid supplements. You will then be monitored with blood pregnancy tests until they are negative. If you have a methotrexate injection, you cannot attempt a pregnancy for three months after treatment. The American College of Obstetricians and Gynecologists recommends that if you proceed with methotrexate, you should avoid the following during treatment:

- Heavy exercise
- Alcohol
- Folic acid
- Nonsteroidals (ibuprofen)
- Prolonged exposure to sun (methotrexate can cause sun sensitivity)

The surgical treatment for an ectopic pregnancy is **operative laparoscopy**, where the doctor either opens the tube (**linear salpingostomy**) or removes the tube (**salpingectomy**). If your blood type is Rh negative, you will need a shot of **Rhogam** after the pregnancy to prevent problems with future pregnancies. Sometime a bigger abdominal incision, laparotomy, is required.

Will I Be Able to Get Pregnant Again?

The chances of a subsequent pregnancy in the uterus are generally good, with rates reported as high as 70%. If you have had more than one ectopic pregnancy, however, the overall success rate of an intrauterine pregnancy is significantly decreased. See the Resources section (page 201) for more detailed statistics on successfully carrying to term after repeated ectopic pregnancies.

Corinna's Story

MY HUSBAND, JEFF, AND I HAVE BEEN TRYING to have a baby for a couple of years. After no success, we found our way to a specialist who told me that one of my tubes was open and one was blocked. On the x-ray, it looked like the dye didn't come out normally on one side. "It pooled," was how the specialist put it.

He suggested I take some pills, Clomid, and time sex. This of course was after he did a number of blood tests and ultrasounds. I took one pill every day for five days, and we had sex at the right time, I think, but I still got my period. This happened repeatedly over two cycles.

The third cycle, I felt different. My breasts were sore, I was peeing a lot, and I was late for my period. I couldn't wait to go to my local pharmacy and get a pregnancy test. I ran home and followed the directions exactly. It said, "Urinate on the stick and look for any color changes." Whoa—it was positive. Excited, I texted my doctor's office. The nurse, who was real nice, said I needed to come in for a blood pregnancy test. The blood test was positive but a low number, so the doctor wanted me to repeat the blood test in two days. I did, and it went up but not enough, so she told me to get a third test. Then I had to get an ultrasound to see the pregnancy. They said it wasn't in my uterus, but it might be too early to detect. I don't remember the exact details, but I remember them saying "pregnancy of unknown location." What does that mean? Pregnancy of unknown location? The nurse said that's the term when they are not sure if it is in the uterus or in my tube. The nurse went on to talk about pain in my abdomen, spotting, and to call if I had really bad pain. Her exact words were "ectopic warnings"; instinctively I hated that term! Days went by. I would go to work, thinking, What if something bad happens and my husband isn't there? Finally, it was just four days from my ultrasound, and I woke up in the middle of the night with unbearable pain. I remembered the nurse said to call day or night. My husband called the doctor, and he said to go right to the emergency room at his hospital.

We got to the ER and were welcomed at the desk. Our doctor had called them, and they were expecting us. They immediately had the ER doctor see me. He looked at my record on the computer and said we need to get a "FAST" bedside ultrasound. It was later that I found out that FAST stands for Focused Assessment with Sonography for Trauma. The ER doctor looked at me and said, "I'm calling your doctor right away." I was in pain, and they started an IV in my arm. I have a high pain tolerance, but this was something else. Then a resident checked my tummy by pressing on it. The pressure made me feel like I was going to jump up and hit the ceiling. She said, "I think you have a ruptured ectopic and we have to take you to the operating room." I could not believe this was happening to me.

My doctor came right away and said they were calling in the OR team. He and the resident doctor explained about the surgery and said they thought they would have to take my tube out. They said they were going in through my belly button, what they called "laparoscopy," but maybe would have to open me up. I was scared, really scared, but then I thought that at least my husband is here and all this didn't happen at work.

In the OR, I remember meeting the anesthesia doctor and I think an anesthetist, too. They made me feel comfortable. Next thing I remember is waking up in the recovery room.

The doctor explained to my husband right after surgery that the tube was ruptured, and my belly was full of blood. He had no choice but to take my tube out since it was "life threatening." I went home that same day, and it took me about a week to get back to myself.

I had to go back to the doctor for a follow-up, and he said my belly incisions were healing well. He said he had to take the one tube that was open out, but I still had two good ovaries and a uterus. To get pregnant in the future, I would need in vitro fertilization (IVF). I asked him why this happened. He looked back at my chart and said that it might have been due to having chlamydia when I was a teenager. My gosh! When I was 19, I had an abnormal Pap. They tested for sexually transmitted diseases and said I had chlamydia. I was prescribed an antibiotic for the infection, and I thought that was the end of it.

Well, we are now saving up for IVF. It's expensive, but if that's what we have to do to have a baby, we'll be ready.

• TAKEAWAY POINTS •

An ectopic pregnancy typically presents with a late period, vaginal bleeding, and abdominal pain.

Prior sexually transmitted infections, even those without symptoms, increase the risk of an ectopic pregnancy.

Prior abdominal/pelvic surgery, especially tubal surgery, increases your risk.

Pregnancy following tubal ligation is likely to be ectopic.

Medical treatment with methotrexate requires that you do not attempt pregnancy for three months following therapy.

• KEY WORDS •

abdominal pain
ectopic pregnancy
human chorionic gonadotropin (HCG)

methotrexate
operative laparoscopy
Rhogam
salpingectomy
sexually transmitted infection
vaginal bleeding

Chapter 14

Help Is Here

Assisted Reproductive Technology

I WAS ALWAYS VERY FOCUSED on my studies. As a senior in high school, I faced a lot of peer pressure to become sexually active. Ultimately, I did have sex with my boyfriend, whom I had been dating for months, on our prom night. We didn't use any birth control. Luckily, my period came on time. Weeks later, though, I was scared that I might have a sexually transmitted infection. I went to a local clinic and sure enough, my test was positive for chlamydia. I never had a symptom. They treated me with a course of antibiotics, and that was seemingly the end of that.

I finished college and law school, got married, and my husband and I decided we wanted to have a child. We were very diligent in coordinating sex with ovulation, month after month. Time marched on and one year later, we were disappointed. No pregnancy. I decided to see my doctor. The doctor did a series of tests that included checking on my tubes. He explained to me that they would do a test by putting dye through the vagina, cervix, and into the uterus and take an x-ray. (This is called a hysterosalpingogram, or HSG.) The HSG was a bit uncomfortable, but I tolerated it okay. I went back to my doctor, and he told me that both of my fallopian tubes were blocked. I was devastated and broke into a sweat. Distraught, I thought, I'll never carry a baby—What will I do? The doctor told me we need to look into in vitro fertilization.—*Molly*

What You Need to Know about IVF

In vitro fertilization (**IVF**) has enabled couples to become parents when previously they had little to no hope. More than 10 million babies have been conceived and born through IVF since Louise Brown, the very first IVF baby, was born in July 1978. Patrick Steptoe and Robert Edwards are credited with this unbelievable process, and in recognition of their ingenuity, they received the Nobel Prize in Physiology or Medicine in 2010.

When Might IVF Be Right for Me?

There are many reasons to proceed with IVF. If one of the scenarios listed below applies to you or your partner, you may be good candidates for in vitro fertilization.

- Tubal factor infertility
- Decreased egg supply
- Male factor infertility
- Unexplained infertility
- Prior tubal ligation
- Fertility preservation prior to cancer therapy

How Does IVF Work?

The Latin term *in vitro* means "in glass," which reflects what happens in the laboratory with an **embryo**. A woman undergoing in vitro fertilization will need a number of preliminary tests that can take one to two cycles to complete. These tests include determining egg supply (ovarian reserve), evaluating the uterine cavity (to determine whether the embryo can easily

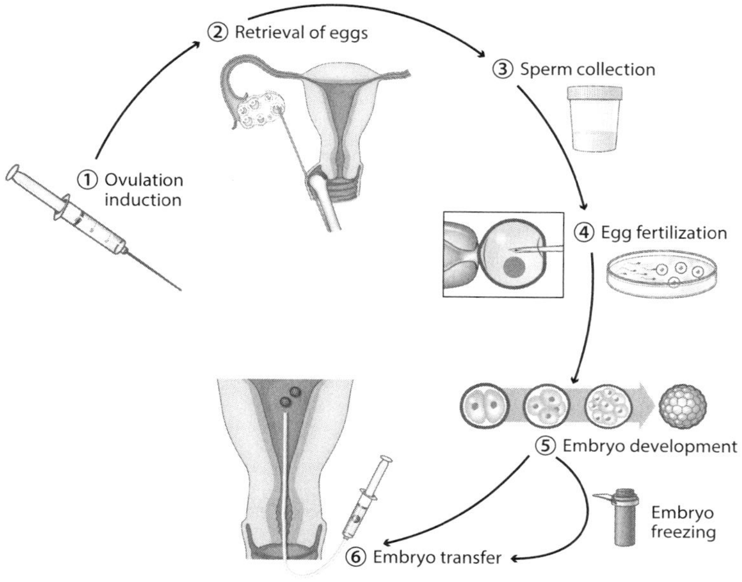

FIGURE 14.5.
Steps of the IVF process.

The placement of an embryo into the uterus is primarily done under ultrasound guidance and requires a full bladder, which provides a "window" through which to see inside the uterus. The ultrasound probe is placed on the abdomen, allowing direct placement of the embryo into the uterine cavity. The patient then continues to use hormones (estrogen and progesterone) to support the pregnancy. The hormones are continued into the end of the first trimester of pregnancy (13 weeks). All the steps involved in in vitro fertilization are shown in figure 14.5.

Success with IVF is partly dependent upon egg supply, maternal age, sperm quality and availability, embryo status, and lifestyle, including obesity, smoking, and alcohol use. Success in large part is focused on the live birth rate and is dependent upon many factors. According to the Society for Assisted Reproductive Technology (SART), the percentage of successful pregnancy ranges from the high 30s to about 50% if the woman is under 35 years of age. For ages 40–41, the success rate is 20%, and over age 42, it is less than 7%.

Women who are 40 or 41 years of age should be evaluated for their ovarian reserve (egg supply) to determine probability of success. You and your health care provider may consider using donor eggs to significantly increase the odds of pregnancy if the ovarian reserve is low. Another option is using a donor embryo, which is like adopting a baby except you carry the pregnancy.

What Are the Complications of IVF?

Complications overall with IVF are rare, but it is important to consider the risks involved. Below is a list of potential complications of IVF treatment.

- Ovarian hyperstimulation syndrome
- Anesthesia-related complications
- Bleeding
- Infection
- Additional surgery
- Cancellation of cycle
- Inability to access the ovary

The most notable of the above complications is **ovarian hyperstimulation syndrome (OHSS)**, which is when the ovaries enlarge. Although rare (it occurs in 3% to 6% of IVF cycles), OHSS may be accompanied by abdominal pain, bloating, nausea, diarrhea, and slight weight gain. It is classified as mild, moderate, or severe. The severe form of OHSS occurs very rarely (in only 0.1% to 2% of cases). Shortness of breath can occur and is more likely with the severe form of OHSS. Complications of OHSS include twisting of an ovary (torsion), ovarian rupture, blood clots (venous thromboembolism), and electrolyte abnormalities. OHSS usually runs its course over one to two weeks and requires monitoring that will be discussed by your doctor; however, severe cases can require hospitalization. Very rarely, blood clots (deep vein thrombosis, or DVT) can occur from fluid shifts out of the bloodstream.

Couples have the option to genetically test an embryo prior to placement into the uterus. This is termed **preimplantation genetic testing (PGT)**. Such tests can identify chromosomal problems such as Down syndrome—this is known as PGT-A (A is for aneuploidy or chromosomal abnormality)—or a specific condition such as cystic fibrosis, which is known as PGT-M (M is for monogenic or single gene). Another test is PGT-SR (SR is for structural rearrangement), which is primarily for patients who have their own chromosomal defects, such as a balanced translocation or deletion/duplication. These tests are not 100% accurate but are reliable. Currently, as a research endeavor, PGT-P (P is for polygenic) provides a risk score for problems that are multifactored, such diabetes, basal cell carcinoma, heart disease, and high blood pressure, but at present this is not available clinically and is experimental.

The bottom line with IVF is that it can indeed result in a baby when no other treatment has been successful. IVF babies are in our opinion true miracles.

April's Story

LET ME TELL YOU ABOUT MY "vanishing good egg supply." I knew we had a problem when month after month came and went and no missed period. We followed the book and timed sex with my ovulation. I always noticed a white vaginal discharge, and the app told us when to do it. I have always had terrible periods—if I could, I would stay in bed, put on the heating pad, and take some pain meds.

My journey begins with my having been diagnosed with endometriosis. I underwent laparoscopy, and I remember after the procedure the doctor told me and my husband that of the four stages of endometriosis, I was a stage 3. I knew that couldn't be good. He went on to say my ovaries were "impacted" by scar tissue. He did the best he could to remove as much as possible. The good news was both my tubes were open. Also, my egg count was good based on the blood tests of my thyroid and uterine lining.

We went to an infertility doctor in the region, and he put me on Clomid. He said even though my husband's sperm count was good, we should do IUIs (intrauterine inseminations) with the Clomid cycles. I ended up with hot flashes and a little dryness with sex, so not my favorite medicine. Once again, cycle after cycle, I got my horrible periods but no pregnancy. We then went with an IVF cycle locally. I got 17 eggs: 7 were "mature," and 5 fertilized. We had decided to do genetic testing on the embryos—they call it PGT for preimplantation genetic testing—and two were normal. We did two fresh embryo transfers, but once again I got my painful periods every time.

Now on to the frozen embryo transfer. I certainly didn't look forward to the full bladder part that was required before each transfer. Anyway, they said the full bladder was necessary to use an ultrasound probe on my belly and know exactly where to place the embryo.

Next, we decided to go with an additional IVF cycle. I took the shots, had the retrieval, and got 12 eggs. One was normal on the PGT testing. We did the embryo transfer, but once again no pregnancy. We followed this with another IVF cycle, got 8 eggs, and unfortunately none of them were mature. I had added acupuncture thinking that might help, but besides relaxing me, it didn't affect the outcome.

So now we are seriously considering donor eggs. One doctor told me, "When the kid cries in the middle of the night, who cares whose egg it is—just take care of the kid." Hmm, interesting advice.

• TAKEAWAY POINTS •

IVF has many indications.

Intracytoplasmic sperm injection (ICSI) can be the best route to fertilization, as is ovulation induction (injections stimulate egg development).

Retrieval is done with a transvaginal probe with twilight anesthesia.

Embryos freeze (cryopreserve) well for a number of years.

The complications of ovarian hyperstimulation (OHSS) often resolve in one to two weeks and are not common.

Preimplantation genetics can identify a genetically normal embryo.

• KEY WORDS •

blastocyst

egg retrieval

embryo

insemination

in vitro fertilization (IVF)

monitored anesthesia care (MAC)

ovarian hyperstimulation syndrome (OHSS)

preimplantation genetic testing (PGT)

tubal factor infertility

Chapter 15

Keep My Eggs Ripe

Social Egg Freezing

I AM 34 YEARS OLD AND have my own national business that I inherited from my dad. My typical day is dedicated to running the business and dealing with getting the best price for goods and services. Over the years I dated several guys, but just never met "Mr. Right." As I look in the mirror, I see a wrinkle or two and one gray hair. I'm aging! One day I would like to have a child of my own, but the thought makes me a bit uncomfortable. I suppose my biological clock is ticking. I am intrigued enough to get on the Internet and begin my search for information about freezing my eggs.—*Michelle*

What You Need to Know about Freezing Your Eggs

The uterus does not age like eggs in the ovary do. Women in their fifties can carry a pregnancy; it would have to be with a fertilized **donor egg**, but it can be done. As women have children later in life, elective egg freezing (sometimes also called **social egg freezing**) is becoming more popular. Many women consider egg freezing to be a form of anxiety prevention and reassurance that having a child is a possibility in the future. Some large corporations that recognize the importance of their employees

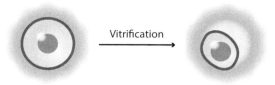

FIGURE 15.1.
Vitrification is the process of preparing an oocyte or embryo for freezing
(cryopreservation).

remaining dedicated to their work while raising families help pay for the cost of egg freezing.

Egg freezing (or oocyte **cryopreservation**, as it is also termed) has become possible owing to advances in in vitro fertilization (IVF). As the largest cell in the body, an egg has a lot of fluid in it called cytoplasm. The process of **vitrification** removes the fluid, shrinks the egg, and allows it to be frozen, or cryopreserved (figure 15.1). Eggs freeze well and stay frozen for a number of years. They require a sperm to be injected (intra-cytoplasmic sperm injection, or ICSI) for fertilization. While egg freezing is by no means a guarantee of a successful liveborn, it increases the odds significantly. The first baby born from a frozen egg (what was called a "vitrification baby") was born in 1986, as reported from Singapore by Dr. Christopher Chen.

Where to Begin?

If you are interested in freezing your eggs, you will first need to see a reproductive endocrinologist, who will take your medical history and do an exam. Then your egg supply will be determined by doing a blood test for **anti-Mullerian hormone (AMH)**. The ideal AMH value is 0.7 ng/ml or higher. Sometimes other tests are done on the third day of the cycle to get a broader picture of egg supply. These blood tests include follicle-stimulating hormone (FSH), luteinizing hormone (LH), and estradiol (E2). An FSH value of 10 or less is ideal, but it varies a bit. The ideal estradiol value is 80 or less, but again it too varies. LH should be about the same as the FSH values. You may need an ultrasound to evaluate your pelvic organs.

How Many Eggs Should Be Frozen?

The number of eggs that you should put into cryopreservation will depend on your age and how many children you plan on having. Online there are **egg freezing calculators** that take these factors into consideration to help you decide how many eggs to freeze:

- Egg Freezing Success Rate Calculator: https://www.fertilitypreservation.org
- Brigham and Women's Hospital Egg Freezing Counseling Tool (EFCT): https://www.mdcalc.com/bwh-egg-freezing-counseling-tool-efct

Some research recommends that women freeze 10 or more eggs. Egg freezing (also known as fertility preservation) should be considered prior to treatment for cancer, as chemotherapy and radiation treatments can negatively affect egg quality.

Importantly, egg freezing is no longer considered experimental, as stated by the American Society for Reproductive Medicine along with the Society for Assisted Reproductive Technology. This decision was made in October 2012.

What's Involved with Egg Freezing?

The tests prior to egg retrieval include obtaining blood for infectious diseases such as hepatitis and HIV. If this is a positive test for one or more of these diseases, then egg storage may require special processing. You may need a transvaginal pelvic ultrasound to determine whether your ovaries are reachable with a needle attached to a vaginal ultrasound probe. The process requires injection of the pituitary hormones (FSH, LH, and other medications) to stimulate the ovary to develop eggs. You will learn how to give yourself the shots. During the injection cycle, several early-morning blood tests of estrogen (estradiol) levels are required. In addition, ultrasound(s) are obtained to visualize the egg (follicle) development. The shots are taken on average for 9–10 days.

The day of egg retrieval, you will arrive at a surgical center and meet the anesthesia team, who will start an IV in your arm. The procedure is done in the surgical center's operating room. Here an anesthetist will give you medication to put you in twilight anesthesia (called conscious sedation or MAC, monitored anesthesia care). The doctor then inserts an ultrasound vaginal probe with a needle while watching an ultrasound monitor that shows the needle and the ovary with the follicles. You do not feel any of this. Each follicle is entered and suctioned (aspirated), but not every follicle has an egg. The fluid obtained from the follicle is immediately handed off to the embryologist in the IVF lab, which is adjacent to the operating room. The embryologist looks under the microscope to determine whether that aspirated follicle has an egg. If so, it is placed in fluid (called egg growth media) in a small petri dish, and then the process of vitrification is done to allow the freezing of the egg. The doctor tries to get every egg that is seen from each ovary. After the process, you will wake up and recover in the recovery room. You can leave the surgical center on the same day, but you may need about a day or so to recover.

The cost of the cycle varies to an extent, so it is best to consult with your IVF team, which should include a financial counselor. In addition to the cost of harvesting your eggs, there is an annual storage fee for the eggs.

When you are ready to carry a pregnancy, the egg is thawed, but not all eggs survive the freeze/thaw cycle, although the vast majority do. The embryologist then requires sperm to be available; you can use your male partner's sperm or donor sperm. The embryologist then assesses the sperm and injects the high-quality sperm into the egg. This is a visual process, and no genetic testing is done. The injected egg is observed for several days, and determination is made whether it can be placed into the uterus or frozen (cryopreserved) for future frozen embryo transfer.

During this time, you will be taking estrogens and progesterone to prepare the lining of your uterus to receive the embryo. Your doctors will monitor the response of the lining of your uterus (endometrium) to the hormones by obtaining a pelvic ultrasound. You may hear the word "trilaminar"; this is an important finding on ultrasound, which indicates a good chance of implantation. The embryo is placed into the uterus under direct ultrasound guidance, which means you need a full bladder just prior to embryo transfer into your uterus. A tiny catheter with a drop of fluid containing the embryo is placed under ultrasound guidance at a targeted spot in the uterine cavity. Immediately after the embryo transfer, you can empty your bladder. You continue on hormones following the embryo transfer through the first trimester of pregnancy. A pregnancy test is obtained soon (about nine days) after the embryo transfer.

Overall, success with IVF is affected by egg quality, embryo quality, as well as the uterus quality, including the lining. Success rates vary in part owing to the age of the egg, when it was frozen, as well as a host of genetic factors within the egg and embryo. Sperm quality is also important.

When it comes to the ideal age for freezing eggs, the sooner the better. At 35 years of age, you are considered to be of advanced maternal age, which implies that there is a slow decrease in egg supply, quality, and the ability for eggs to get fertilized and progress accordingly. Hence it is a good idea to freeze your eggs before the age of 35.

If you are told you have "decreased ovarian reserve," which means you are heading toward early menopause, but still have oocytes, it becomes even more important to freeze your eggs before the egg supply is no longer available. Some couples, more often for religious reasons, prefer to inseminate a limited number of eggs that would have the potential to become embryos and freeze the remaining eggs.

Using donor eggs is an option should you not have your own (autologous) eggs available for fertilization and pregnancy. Donor egg banks carefully screen donors and will provide information about them so that you can make the right decision for you.

There does not appear to be any increase in chromosomal abnormalities, birth defects, or developmental defects in babies born with frozen eggs, compared to baseline abnormalities. Risks do occur, although they are not common. One risk is ovarian hyperstimulation syndrome (OHSS). In OHSS, the ovaries enlarge, and there is abdominal bloating and to some degree discomfort as pain in the abdomen occurs. Sometimes, blood clots (deep vein thrombosis, or DVT) can occur from fluid shifts out of the bloodstream, but this is very rare. Other risks with IVF are essentially those with any surgical procedure and include bleeding, infection, and anesthesia-related problems. But in healthy women, these problems are rare. For more information on the risks of IVF, see chapter 14.

Danica's Story

ONE MORNING I WOKE UP and the realization hit me that I had turned 35. I said to myself, Hmm, I'm not getting any younger. I don't have Mr. Right on my radar screen right now, but one day I want to have children. I love kids and want a bunch of my own. What options do I have? My life is my career. I am a bank manager for a large regional bank, and while they provide excellent health insurance, they do not cover the cost of egg freezing. So I went online, Instagram to be exact, and got helpful information. I looked at several centers, but it looks expensive, like $15,000. I do have some money saved up, so I can afford the expense. I ended up looking at a number of websites for IVF centers and liked the one at a major medical center here in town.

I mustered up enough courage to call and make an appointment. Well, the day arrived. The doctor could not have been nicer, and said he understood exactly why I wanted to freeze my eggs. He spent an hour with me talking about tests to see if I had enough eggs—I think he called it my ovarian reserve. Then I needed an ultrasound to see if they could get to my ovaries. He gave me statistics and numbers and said that ideally we would freeze at least 10 eggs, but we can calculate the right number based on how many children I plan to have. The office staff made me feel welcome and comfortable. They told me to feel free to call or email them with any questions. I felt empowered that I was now in charge of my own future fertility. I recalled the song by Helen Reddy, "I Am Woman."

So all the tests were done and I again met with the doctor, this time by telemedicine. He said my egg supply was good, and he thought there should be no problem getting to my ovaries. Whew, what a relief. I knew I had to give myself shots every day for about nine days, and I was told to plan on coming in the office real early every day for a blood test to see how my ovaries were responding. I felt my body react to these medicines. I was a bit bloated and constipated, but they told me to take a stool softener. The doctors explained that this was due to the hormone changes from the shots.

Finally, the day to get the eggs out came. I went to the IVF center and met the anesthesia folks, who were reassuring and made me feel comfortable. My best friend Sarah drove me to the IVF center and back home afterward. They started an IV in my arm, and then we went to the operating room, where they took the eggs out. I noticed an ultrasound machine and I asked what it was for. They said it was for the doctor to see the ovaries and the location of the eggs as they retrieved them. I woke up in the recovery room. The doctor came over and said it went well. In all, we got 12 eggs. This was a different doctor than the one I first saw.

I was half-awake in the recovery room and they said they were going to freeze all 12 eggs because they all were mature. I think they mentioned something about taking the water out of each egg; I think they called it "vitrification" or something like that. I don't really remember. Sarah took me home, and I slept most of the day. The next day I stayed home, although I felt fine. I remember them saying the eggs stay frozen a long time, like five or more years.

Well wouldn't you know it, two years later Mr. Right, now my husband, shows up on the scene. Now I am 37 years old. Of course, we talked about having a baby. I went back to that same doctor I visited two years back. He ran a blood test and said my egg supply was bad. I thought to myself, How can that happen? Two years ago it was fine. We had been trying to have a baby for six months at that point. Thankfully, because I had my frozen eggs, we have options to get pregnant. The doctor and I talked about how they could thaw the egg and inject one of my husband's sperm into it. We did just that, and then they put one embryo into my uterus. I wasn't a happy camper that day because I needed a full bladder so they would know exactly where in my uterus to put the embryo, and then I had to put progesterone pills in my vagina three times a day. Although I was concerned the pills would fall out, I was reassured that they were safely in my vagina. I prayed for it to work since I was not sure if we could afford another IVF cycle. While we were waiting for the embryologist to bring the embryo to place in my uterus, I kept thinking if we would be good parents. Well, lo and behold, the pregnancy test was positive. Nine months later, Tucker, my adorable little guy, arrived. We love him like you can't begin to imagine.

• TAKEAWAY POINTS •

Egg freezing is a good option allowing a woman to carry a pregnancy when she wishes.

Egg calculators address patient age and number of planned children.

Following preliminary tests, hormone injections for 9 to 10 days are required for ovarian egg development.

The eggs are removed via a needle attached to a transvaginal probe.

Twilight anesthesia is used to harvest eggs.

Fertilization requires sperm injection into the egg.

Egg freezing is a good option for cancer patients, prior to treatment.

• KEY WORDS •

anti-Mullerian hormone (AMH)
cryopreservation
donor egg
egg freezing calculators
social egg freezing
vitrification

Chapter 16

Cancer Can't Stop Me

Fertility Preservation

I'M 16 YEARS OLD AND a junior in high school. I run track and get mostly As with an occasional B. I like to think I'm popular, and my friends are frequently seeking my advice. I have always been in excellent health, but recently I noticed I'm tired and can't run as far or as fast as I used to. I noticed a lump in my neck while clasping a necklace. It became painful, and I started to run a low-grade fever, around 100.3. Weight loss followed soon after, with excessive sweating. On occasion I am short of breath when walking up the stairs and prone to frequent colds. Because this never happened before, my mom suggested I see our primary care provider. The doctor ran several tests and concluded that I have non-Hodgkin lymphoma. When we got the news, Mom looked painfully upset as tears poured out of her eyes. Devastated by the news, my fears about the cancer treatment deepened because I learned in school that cancer treatment can make you sterile. The doctor suggested I see a reproductive endocrinologist to preserve my eggs so that one day I can hopefully have my own (genetic) child. The PCP talked about "life after cancer." The suggestion of having my own child one day relieved a little of the anxiety placed upon my shoulders.—*Mia*

What You Need to Know about Cancer and Fertility

As progress in cancer treatment advances and five-year survival rates are ever increasing, future fertility can become a reality. **Fertility preservation** is far-reaching, with the ability to freeze (cryopreserve) eggs (oocytes) or ovarian tissue for women and sperm or testicular tissue for men. These efforts are all focused on allowing an individual to one day have their own genetic child.

In Mia's case, the journey started with a blood test for her egg supply. This was followed by an ultrasound to look at her ovaries and uterus. The cancer specialist, called an oncologist, usually gives a small window, perhaps two to four weeks, to take medications to stimulate the ovaries to develop a number of eggs. This requires shots, usually under the skin (subcutaneous), of the pituitary hormones, with careful and frequent blood test monitoring. One to two pelvic ultrasounds are usually included to visualize the ovaries and the developing follicles. The injections on average go on for 9 to 10 days. The taking of eggs (retrieval) is done while under twilight anesthesia, also called conscious sedation or monitored anesthesia care (MAC). An ultrasound probe placed in the vagina has a needle that enters the ovary, and each follicle is aspirated with the hope it has an egg. The egg is processed in such a way as to remove the high water content, a process called vitrification, which allows eggs to be frozen, or cryopreserved. The eggs freeze well in general, and can be preserved for a number of years.

When the patient wants to become pregnant and carry the baby, it requires a sperm to be injected into the egg through a process called ICSI, which stands for intracytoplasmic sperm injection. We call this insertion of the sperm into the egg "insemination." Once fertilization occurs, the egg is now an embryo, which is placed into the uterus that has a prepared lining. The latter is accomplished by putting the patient on estrogens and progesterone before embryo transfer. The embryo is placed into the uterus under direct ultrasound guidance, which requires a full bladder immediately prior to transferring the embryo; embryo transfer is the term for placing the embryo into the uterus.

If the patient has a male partner, then his sperm can be used to inseminate the egg and create an embryo. Embryos freeze extremely well, five or more years on average. It is important to understand that not every egg or embryo survives the freeze/thaw cycle, but the good news is the vast majority do.

If a girl has cancer and the oncologist does not think a **fast-track IVF cycle** to preserve eggs is acceptable, the patient may qualify for ovarian tissue **cryopreservation** before chemo or **radiation therapy**. Here the specialist, a gynecologic surgeon, removes an entire ovary, which is usually done using a laparoscope during minimally invasive surgery. The fertility preservation team then freezes the ovary, usually in a number of segments, each in its own straw, and places it in liquid nitrogen ($-196°$C) for freezing and preserving the ovarian tissue until it is ready to be utilized. Sometimes the ovarian tissue can be returned to its normal location adjacent to the fallopian tube and uterus in the hopes that it works again, and many times it does, thus allowing pregnancy to occur through sexual intercourse. Sometimes in vitro fertilization (IVF) is required.

Research continues to explore the potential of eggs from the ovarian tissue that have been matured in a laboratory being able to receive sperm for ICSI. This egg maturing process is known as **in vitro maturation**. The first baby born from "vitrified warmed human eggs" injected with sperm was reported in 1999.

We use the term oncofertility to reflect the blending of the cancer part (oncology) with the fertility part (primarily reproductive endocrinology) (figure 16.1). Much progress has been made regarding fertility preservation as it relates to cancer treatment in part because of the efforts of the National Institutes of Health and National Cancer Institute to assist in developing a consortium of several major medical centers. Teams have

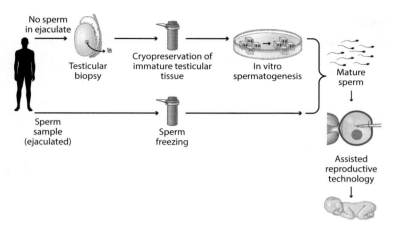

FIGURE 16.1.
Oncofertility: a preservation process (male).

been developed at major medical centers, and care is provided from pediatric age on up. Research is also advancing regarding stem cells and the potential to channel the cell into becoming an egg (oocyte) or sperm.

If the uterus is unaffected by cancer treatment but no eggs become available, a pregnancy can be achieved with donor eggs. **Egg banks** worldwide make donor eggs available to women who desire to pursue this option. Here again, one sperm is injected into one egg for fertilization, and the resulting embryo is transferred into the cancer-free patient's uterus.

Men who face a cancer diagnosis and want to preserve their fertility may freeze their sperm for future use. Ejaculated sperm freeze well. In one case, a pregnancy resulted from sperm frozen for 22 years. If you wish to pursue this option, you should let your health care provider know before starting cancer treatment.

Cancer Treatment Drugs That Affect Eggs and Sperm

Listed below are cancer therapy drugs based on their risk of causing infertility. The high-risk treatments are more likely to result in permanent fertility impairment in comparison to the other categories. Age of onset, type of cancer, and treatment doses also influence the effect of the **chemotherapy** agent. It is hard to predict the specific effect of the chemotherapeutic agent on future fertility, so you should speak with your prescribing provider about up-to-date information.

High-Risk Category
- Busulfan
- Chlorambucil
- Chlormethine
- Cyclophosphamide
- Ifosamide
- Melphalan
- Procarbazine

Medium-Risk Category
- Doxorubicin
- Platinum analogs (Cisplatin and Carboplatin)

Low-Risk Category
- Bleomycin
- Dactinomycin
- 5-Floururacil
- Mercaptopurine
- Methotrexate
- Vinblastine
- Vincristine

Francine's Story

I WAS 19 YEARS OLD and noted something on my neck was irritated by the turtleneck blouse I was wearing. I reached in and felt a lump. I didn't think much of it at the moment. I had experienced a bad cold a week earlier and thought that perhaps the two were related. Well, two weeks later, I noticed that the lump had gotten bigger. Oh boy, I thought, Now what? I called my mom about it, and she said, "As soon as you are home for the holidays, we are going to the doctor."

Our family doctor took one look at me, checked the lump, and said that I needed to see a specialist. We wound up at a big local cancer center. I was shaking as we met with the doctor. She was very nice and tried to calm me down while my mom held my hand the entire time. The doctor felt the lump and said that I would need to get some tests done right away. The doctor, now with her team in the room, said I needed a PET (positron emission tomography) scan and some blood work. She ordered a biopsy of the lump and explained to me that a needle would go into the lump and then the biopsy would be sent to the pathologist. We left her office feeling we had a plan, but I was trembling, with all kinds of thoughts rushing through my mind—What if, what if, is all I could think of.

The doctor's office called and asked me to return to the office now that my tests were back. I was so scared that I could hardly get myself dressed that day. My mom drove, and when we pulled into the parking lot, I asked my mom, "What if it's cancer?" She said, "Now, let's just see what the doctor says. There's no sense getting all worked up about it." I wiped the tears from my eyes.

While waiting in the doctor's office, I could not keep my knees from trembling and my eyes from welling up. The doctor came in and showed us the report's diagnosis: Hodgkin lymphoma. Then I remember she said, "classic type" and something about "nodular." She said it affects younger people, like 15- to 35-year-olds. Through the haze of my diagnosis, I can only recall the doctor saying that I would need chemotherapy.

My mom asked, "Will she ever be able to have a baby?" The doctor said maybe, if I could quickly get to a specialist who deals with such cases. The cancer doctor (oncologist) said that the medicines and chemotherapy would probably wipe out my chance of having my own baby. I kept sobbing, thinking to myself, No baby ever! The doctor said that we need to see another doctor, a reproductive endocrinology and infertility specialist. I thought, Infertility? I'm not trying to get pregnant; why would we want to see that doctor? Frankly, I was getting tired of doctors.

This doctor was very thoughtful and spent a lot of time with us. She told us we could quickly do some tests to see if I had eggs. She said usually we could proceed with taking shots to stimulate my ovaries to make eggs, then take them out while I was kind of out of it, and freeze the eggs until I was cured. Later I could put an embryo in my uterus. She said a second option was to have one of my ovaries removed, frozen, and then in the future placed back inside my body or see if we can get eggs from the ovarian tissue. He said that the latter was a bit more complicated in that there is a maturing process (in vitro maturation) in the lab. If I have eggs, they would inject a sperm and put the baby—called an embryo—in my uterus. But all of this depended on the oncologist giving us the okay to do this before they started chemotherapy. My head was spinning with all the information!

The doctor called the oncologist while I was in her office. She kept saying, "Okay. Sounds good; let me talk to her." She said we got the go-ahead for either taking the shots, getting my eggs out, or surgery to remove one of my ovaries. I quickly talked to my mom, and we decided to try saving my eggs. The doctor said we should freeze my eggs; she used the word "cryopreserve." She said eggs freeze well, for a number of years, but it would require injecting a sperm into each egg when I was ready to become pregnant.

After doing the tests, the infertility doctor called me to say that I had a good egg supply, and we could begin the process immediately. I went through the whole procedure as directed, including my shots every day, and then I went to the center, where we got 14 eggs.

I went back to the oncologist, and she proceeded with the medicine for Hodgkin lymphoma. I lost all my beautiful hair, but eventually it grew back. Thank heavens! As I look back, the whole cancer team was great, and I felt they were always there for me.

Now I am two years out, cancer-free so far. Pray for me and my eggs.

• TAKEAWAY POINTS •

Research is ongoing, and there is hope for fertility following cancer treatment. It is strongly encouraged that you discuss the options with your oncologist early in your diagnosis in order to maximize the chances of having your own biological child.

The following can be frozen (cryopreserved):

- o eggs (oocytes)
- o embryos
- o ovarian tissue
- o sperm
- o testicular tissue

• KEY WORDS •

chemotherapy
cryopreservation
egg bank
fast-track IVF cycle
fertility preservation
in vitro maturation
radiation therapy

Chapter 17

Building a Nontraditional Family

Nonbinary Fertility

I ALWAYS FELT A BIT DIFFERENT as I was growing up. I liked to play with toy soldiers and toy guns. I was called a "tomboy" and sometimes dressed like a boy. Time progressed, and I really felt uncomfortable in my body. So, I decided as a teenager to muster up the courage to talk to my doctor about these feelings. He was great, listened carefully, and made me feel really comfortable. He suggested that I have a behavioral health evaluation. He told me about gender dysphoria, which he defined as "feelings of distress due to a strong desire to be of another gender than the one assigned at birth." It was such a relief to have found someone to listen to me and understand me. The doctor also suggested I see a team of health care providers that dealt with people who are transgender. The team included a pediatric endocrinologist who discussed taking male hormones, testosterone, to allow me to transition to a male. That doctor also suggested I freeze my eggs (oocytes) so that one day I could have my own genetic child. Events progressed, and I received a number of injections to stimulate my ovaries. Then my eggs were removed under ultrasound guidance while I was in twilight anesthesia. The eggs were preserved for the future. I went on to have masculinizing surgery, and the medical term "transman" was used to describe me, a transgender male.—*Shania*

What You Need to Know about Fertility Preservation

Medical care for transgender patients involves physical alteration or transition to the opposite sex. This includes hormone treatment as well as genital surgery for sex reassignment. Fertility treatment for transgender patients involves the preservation of sperm or eggs (oocytes) for future fertilization and assurance of having one's own genetic child. The timing of this treatment is extremely important, since cross-sex hormones can interfere with successful preservation of what are termed "gametes" (sperm or eggs).

The World Professional Association for Transgender Health and the Endocrine Society recommend fertility counseling prior to hormonal therapy. The **multidisciplinary approach** includes adolescent medicine specialists, psychologists, endocrinologists both pediatric and reproductive, and surgeons with expertise in genital reconstruction. A psychiatrist may also be required to address associated mental health issues, or comorbidities, which can affect the final outcome. Parental involvement is important for adolescents going through treatment.

Important Terminology

The below terms are often used to describe aspects of the transgender experience. For more information, refer to the *DSM-5* (*Diagnostic and Statistical Manual of Mental Disorders*, fifth edition).

Body dysmorphia: Distress caused by dissatisfaction with one's physical body.

Gender-affirming hormone therapy: The use of hormones (testosterone and estrogen) to transition to the desired sex.

Gender dysphoria: Distress caused by having a body that does not match one's gender identity.

Transgender: A person whose gender identity does not match the sex assigned at birth.

Transman: Female to male transgender person.

Transwoman: Male to female transgender person.

Options for Preserving Fertility

The options for **fertility preservation** will differ depending on whether you are a transgender woman (table 17.1) or transgender man (table 17.2).

TABLE 17.1.
Options for transgender women

Sperm banking	If post-pubertal
Sperm aspiration from testicle	If post-pubertal
Testicular tissue freezing	If pre-pubertal

TABLE 17.2.
Options for transgender men

Egg (oocyte) freezing	If post-pubertal
Embryo freezing	If has male partner or donor sperm
Ovarian tissue freezing	If pre-pubertal (rare)

Transgender men who wish to have their own biological children will need to have their eggs retrieved and cryopreserved before getting pregnant (chapters 14 and 15). Transgender women would need to have their sperm collected and then frozen for future use (chapter 17). For all transgender patients hoping to become parents in the future, the timing of fertility preservation is important. A suggested sequence is as follows:

1. Diagnosis and desired sex assignment
2. Discussion of fertility preservation options
3. Discussion of the required hormone treatment for fertility preservation
4. Proceed with sperm or egg preservation
5. Begin medical hormonal treatment for transition to the opposite sex
6. Sex reassignment surgery, if desired

Considerations for Transgender Parents

Transgender men (transmen) can carry a pregnancy to term, but doing so should be carefully considered for a number of reasons, especially psychological and social ones. There may be challenges for transmen that are beyond physical and biological barriers. Surrogacy and adoption are alternative options for carrying a pregnancy, but both of these routes to parenthood are expensive. Assistance in finding a surrogate is available through a number of agencies online. Growinggenerations.com, giftto lifesurrogacy.com, surrogate.com, and genesisrising.com can provide additional information.

Social stigma and discrimination against transgender patients exist in the health care system, so it is ideal to have a team of professionals that includes health care providers and legal experts who can help guide you through the process of having a child. For example, the fertility preservation option is not always suggested to transgender patients prior to hormonal therapy, even though more than half of transmen desire their own genetic child.

Current research shows that having a transgender parent does not affect a child's gender identity or sexual orientation. Public opinion supports health care providers assisting transgender patients to have their own biological child.

The World Professional Association for Transgender Health and the Endocrine Society provide guidelines and other information on transgender parents for health care professionals. One of the key points of the association and society is making individuals aware of future fertility options. Understanding the consequences of hormone therapy is also important, as there may be negative health effects from the long-term use of cross-sex hormones. The World Professional Association for Transgender Health (WPATH) can provide the latest information on research in this area.

Bryson's Story

I ALWAYS FELT like I should be a boy since I reached puberty. When I was a child, I never liked playing with dolls. I always wanted a bow and arrow or to play "shoot 'em up." I gravitated to hanging out with the boys and really never had a girlfriend that I could confide in growing up. I knew something must not be right with me. I remember my pediatrician telling my mom not to worry because I'd grow out of it. Now, well into my teens, I read an article on transmen and thought to myself, That's me! I had the courage to bring it up with my pediatrician when we met one on one. She suggested I see a pediatric endocrinologist and set me up with a team that included a psychologist and a surgeon who deals with transgender patients. The endocrinologist suggested, after all my tests were completed, that I consider storing my eggs so that one day I could have my own genetic child. She called it "your own biological child."

I was referred to a reproductive endocrinologist. He and his team were great, and they made me feel comfortable. But I must say sitting in the waiting room with all these women made me a bit queasy. I didn't like the medical assistant who asked me all these questions and looked at me as if to say, "What are you doing here?" I thought she was insensitive to say the least. I told the reproductive endocrinologist I wanted to start testosterone, but the pediatric endocrinologist thought I should first freeze my eggs. Wow, what a relief to have a "road map" of what I could do to one day have my own child. Now we were getting somewhere! There was discussion that I would need a hysterectomy, but that would be a bit down the road. This would be followed by what they called "reconstructive surgery" to change my female parts into male parts. I was game!

The process for egg freezing began. It seemed like there were so many tests. They had to determine if I had enough eggs, so they did a blood test and an ultrasound to check my female parts. Then the nurse instructed me how to give myself shots under the skin of the actual pituitary hormones to stimulate my ovaries to develop and mature my eggs. They said it would take 9 or 10 days. Then I was told I would be asleep, under twilight anesthesia, and an ultrasound probe would be placed in my vagina. A needle would be placed from the vagina into each of my ovaries to take out the eggs. Well, what do you know. They retrieved 15 eggs. I call them my little "ice cubes"; they are there when I am ready to use them.

I learned about a program called SprOUT Family, which is a nonprofit for LGBTQ folks like me. They provide great information including centers that deal with transgender patients. I would venture to guess there are a lot of transgender folks who don't know you can freeze your eggs or your sperm early on. Personally, I don't think there is enough discussion about "family building options" for LGBTQ individuals, and that is unfortunate. I understand that once you start the hormones, testosterone in my case, it can have a bad impact on getting eggs. Once I have the surgery, in essence I am sterilized and lose any chance to have my own biological kid. I'll be looking for a gestational carrier (surrogate) a bit down the road.

• TAKEAWAY POINTS •

Transgender patients should consider fertility preservation prior to transition.

A multidisciplinary team approach works best.

Consider sperm or egg freezing prior to medical treatment.

Explore options for carrying a pregnancy.

• **KEY WORDS** •

body dysmorphia
fertility preservation
gender dysphoria
multidisciplinary approach
transgender

Chapter 18

Building a Family While Serving the Nation

Military Fertility Services

I'VE BEEN ON ACTIVE DUTY for eight years, and in this time not once have I been able to get pregnant. Traveling and being on duty is stressful as it is, but it makes having a baby real challenging. To date we have undergone an in vitro fertilization (IVF) cycle while in the military and have eight frozen embryos. I was deployed twice, and now we are ready to have a family. I have been stationed in the state of Washington, and my embryos are stored at a civilian location in Arizona. When I had the preliminary tests prior to my embryo transfer, it was noted that I have fibroids in the lining of my uterus. I decided to get care from a major military facility that offered me surgical treatment of my fibroids. The procedure was a hysteroscopic myomectomy, in which the fibroids in the lining of the uterus were "shaved down" in the location where the baby will grow. I had an ultrasound following the surgery, and the uterine lining was good to go for an embryo transfer. They shipped my embryos to the local IVF facility where I am stationed. I'm going to have an embryo transfer within the next two months.—*Amelia*

What You Need to Know about Military Infertility Services

Where you go to access infertility services depends on your current status in the military. If you are on active duty, you or your dependent should contact the **TRICARE** benefits office or your **primary care manager (PCM)**. If you are a veteran, you may qualify for health care through the US Department of Veterans Affairs (VA) hospital system; for detailed eligibility requirements, you should visit the VA Health Benefits website (https://www.va.gov/health-care/about-va-health-benefits/). Since the **VA hospital system** and the (active) military are separate entities, it means there are separate tracks to pursue. Not all veterans may be entitled to care at the VA, and unless an active-duty member retires from the military, they will not be entitled to military health care after leaving active duty.

What Factors Can Influence My Fertility While on Active Duty?

Serving in the military can affect both your ability to get pregnant and the health of your pregnancy. There are some steps you can take to prepare yourself for pregnancy as well as to protect yourself and your pregnancy while on active duty.

Lifestyle

Lifestyle choices are key to any healthy pregnancy. Be sure to eat a balanced diet, exercise regularly, and address medical issues while you're on active military service. It's also a good idea to start taking a prenatal vitamin that contains folic acid and to avoid alcohol, drugs, and tobacco. For information on preconception counseling, see chapter 2.

Toxins

You may be concerned about potential exposure to environmental toxins while on active duty. Certain toxins—ionizing radiation, inorganic lead, Agent Orange, and other environmental toxins—can adversely affect the male reproductive tract.

Emotional and Physical Trauma

Deployment can pose challenges for military personnel as well as their partners. Stress on the relationship can be an additional problem that could result in impotence or affect ovulation. Trauma experienced in the course of duty, including extensive genital and perineal wounds, can significantly affect the sperm count of the male reproductive tract.

How Can I Optimize My Chances of a Pregnancy?

More details about **optimizing fertility** can be found in chapter 2. If you are planning to get pregnant, you should work with your health care provider to take the following steps.

- Eat a nutritious diet; take folic acid supplements; and stop smoking, drinking alcohol, or using drugs.
- Undergo pre-pregnancy testing (semen analysis, ovarian reserve testing).
- Verify that you are up to date with all recommended vaccinations.
- Ensure the medications you are taking do not have possible adverse effects on pregnancy.
- Work to manage any chronic medical conditions.

I Have an Infertility Diagnosis. Where Do I Go for Treatment?

If you are a veteran, it is important to discuss your options with your local VA hospital provider. The Serving Our Veterans Program partners with local **civilian fertility centers** and provides discounts for veterans. If you are an active military member, work with your PCM at a military treatment center. Some military facilities, in conjunction with civilian partners, deliver a large range of infertility services (table 18.1). At this time, these sites include:

- Walter Reed National Military Medical Center in Bethesda, Maryland

TABLE 18.1.

Military infertility programs and annual reported IVF statistics (in percentages)

INFERTILITY PROGRAMS	IVF LIVE BIRTH RATES PER EGG RETRIEVAL
Nationwide	46.7
Brooke Army Medical Center	44.8
Madigan Army Medical Center	54.2
Tripler Army Medical Center	42.6
Walter Reed Medical Center	43.8

Note: Statistics vary depending on year of reporting. Reported to the Society for Assisted Reproductive Technology (SART).

- Tripler Army Medical Center in Honolulu, Hawaii
- Womack Army Medical Center in Tacoma, Washington
- San Antonio Military Medical Center in San Antonio, Texas
- Naval Medical Center in San Diego, California

What Are My Treatment Options?

Treatment can range from medical to surgical options; see chapter 3 for details. The military participates in assisted reproductive technology (IVF) and if medically indicated, the plans provide coverage for egg or embryo freezing and storage. The US Centers for Disease Control and Prevention (CDC) reported that in one year, more than 1,400 IVF cycles were provided to the military. This included egg freezing as well as the military personnel undergoing embryo freezing for the future and resulted in more than 400 pregnancies and deliveries (Peck, 2019). For more information on the statistics for individual infertility programs, visit the website of the Society for Assisted Reproductive Technology (www.sart.org).

What about Financial Support for Infertility Services?

The cost for assisted reproductive technologies can leave one feeling overwhelmed and unsure whether it's affordable. The good news is that military benefits include IVF and other fertility treatments.

VHA Directive 1332 established VA medical benefits to include infertility services, including diagnosis and specific treatment options. You can find more details regarding eligibility and the prerequisites for qualifying for such services by contacting the Women Veterans Call Center (855-829-6636).

Additionally, RESOLVE is a national infertility association with resources that may be beneficial to military personnel. RESOLVE can help you determine the best avenue for you with regard to what fertility services are covered by the military. The Military Officers Association of America (MOAA) is another key advocate for veteran and active military members.

The Health Care Fairness for Military Act of 2021 expanded TRICARE eligibility for adults up to 26 years of age. TRICARE insurance may cover basic fertility evaluation and possibly treatment. The following are common diagnostic tests that should be covered by TRICARE insurance:

- Semen analysis
- Ovarian reserve testing
- Other hormonal testing
- Genetic (chromosomal) studies
- Immunologic tests
- Infectious agent assessment related to infertility

The following treatment options may not be covered by TRICARE:

- Artificial or intrauterine insemination
- Donor sperm
- Reversal of sterilization
- Erectile dysfunction from psychological causes:
  o depression treatment
  o anxiety treatment
  o stress management
- In vitro fertilization

- Fertility preservation
- Surrogacy
- Prescription medications to treat ovulation or male infertility (determined on a case-by-case basis)

It is possible that TRICARE pays for segments of treatment care, and what is not covered becomes an out-of-pocket expense. If you are an active-duty member experiencing infertility due to a serious injury or illness sustained while serving in the military, it is possible that you can obtain special coverage. Based upon a 2017 Supplemental Health Care Program, benefits were extended to include "while on active duty" and "a new diagnosis of cancer" affecting future fertility. For example, in 2019, *Military Families Magazine* provided information for military personnel, reporting that TRICARE may pay for IVF if an active member is "seriously or severely injured" or experiences "loss of natural procreative ability."

Congress and Infertility in the Military: Current Initiative

Congresswoman Marilyn Strickland (WA-10) introduced a bill that proposes expanding access to fertility care for servicemembers and dependents. It would expand TRICARE coverage for assisted reproductive technology / IVF services for all active-duty service members. As of late 2022, the bill is proceeding through Congress.

Rori's Story

I WAS ACTIVE DUTY for four years and then became a civilian. We have traveled the world. We went to try to have a baby and were interrupted by Ben being deployed. We had trouble timing sex with my ovulation. We tried for what seemed like an eternity. I knew we hit the right time at least six times (cycles) one year and nothing. What do I do; where do I turn? I went to the local VA and saw the general medical officer, and they couldn't have been more helpful. We were able to get a sperm count when Ben was in the states, and thank God he was okay. The doctor was great and said we needed to run a few tests and come up with a treatment plan. The doctor talked about Clomid because my cycles started to be irregular. I took the pills for five days, and thank heavens Ben was in town. We had sex daily for several days, and then I felt kind of funny. My breasts were sore, I was peeing all the time, and then I felt like I needed to throw up every day. I went back to the VA for a blood test, and guess what? It was positive. I can't thank the VA docs enough for making it happen! Olivia is the best thing that ever happened to us.

• TAKEAWAY POINTS •

The military has infertility coverage benefits.

Whether you are active military or a veteran dictates where you can receive care for infertility services.

Check with your insurance policy regarding infertility coverage.

Explore major military health centers for available fertility treatment services.

• KEY WORDS •

civilian fertility centers
deployment
optimizing fertility
primary care manager (PCM)
TRICARE
VA hospital system
VHA Directive 1332

REFERENCE

Peck, Andrea D. 2019. "IVF Helps Military Couples Grow Families." *Military Families Magazine*, August 22, 2019. https://militaryfamilies .com/military-health/ivf-helps-military-couples-grow-families/.

Chapter 19

Help Me Preserve My Sanity

Managing Stress

DOC, YOU NEED TO HELP ME. My wife is obsessed with getting pregnant, but we have several problems. One, she is older (42 years old), and two, she has fibroids in her uterus. She tells me how her periods have become irregular, although in the past they were like clockwork every month. My real concern is she has painted our spare bedroom, purchased a crib, and bought baby clothes. I'm a bit older, too (50 years old), and we have a great marriage, but this is the one thing she stresses about all day long. What should we do?—*Ahmed*

What You Need to Know about Stress

Let's begin with a definition. The *Oxford Dictionary* defines **stress** as "a state of mental or emotional stress or tension secondary to adverse or very demanding circumstances." Stress is frequently associated with the body producing hormones (cortisol) to cope with the problem. A person's reaction to stress is sometimes called the "fight-or-flight response."

Stress can lead to infertility by causing your menstrual cycles to be irregular or sometimes to stop completely. In some cases, stress can bring isolation from family and friends, thus leading to an escalating or "snow-ball" effect. We must acknowledge that the opposite is also true: infertility causes stress. Infertility is associated with depression, anxiety, isolation, and loss of control. It is especially a concern for patients with recurrent miscarriages. Post-traumatic stress disorder (PTSD) has also been reported with the stress of infertility. Infertility is often a **silent struggle**, as described by a neuroscience publication (Rooney and Domar, 2018).

How Is Stress Evaluated?

Evaluation of stress is based on the seriousness of the problem. You should be encouraged to speak with someone, ideally a health care professional, especially if it is affecting your life. Stress scales such as the Perceived Stress Scale or the COMPI Fertility Problems Stress Scale can help evaluate the level of stress you are experiencing. The results of these scales are then addressed by a health care professional and used especially in the diagnostic stage.

It is important to determine whether stress has affected your menstrual cycle or ovulation and to address this possibility with your doctor or advanced practice provider (APP).

How Do You Treat the Many Causes of Stress?

There are varied approaches to **addressing stress**. It may begin with discussing your stress and anxiety with your partner or significant other. As a couple, you may well arrive at a solution. **Alternative therapies**—yoga, aromatherapy, relaxation, select herbal preparations, chiropractic therapy, biofeedback, meditation, cognitive behavioral therapy—may also help alleviate stress. Individual and group therapy as well as mind/body programs are other options for addressing infertility-related stress.

Scientific studies have found acupuncture to be a beneficial treatment. A type of Chinese medicine, acupuncture focuses on an energy source called *qi*, which practitioners believe is integrally involved with overall health. In theory, *qi* moves throughout the body much like blood is propelled through the circulatory system, but it travels via lines known as meridians. Stress can disturb this flow of *qi*. In acupuncture, needles are inserted at specific pressure points to allow restoration of *qi* balance, and some studies attest to overall improvement in body health. Needles are placed millimeters away from specific nerves. The theory is that the nervous system then produces analgesic (painkilling) chemicals that have a positive effect on the brain. Individuals feel more balanced and in control following acupuncture, and in some cases experience a decrease in the body's production of cortisol. Results are usually rapid.

Suggestions for Coping with the Stress of Infertility

If you are feeling stressed by the challenges of infertility, you might consider one or more of the following coping strategies.

- Acknowledge that you are stressed.
- It's okay to grieve, cry, or even be angry about it.
- Try to focus on the present and the future, not the past.
- Seek support in others who have experienced infertility.
- Communicate with your partner or significant other.
- Change your mindset; by pursuing a strategy of cognitive restructuring, you may be able to reframe your attitude in a positive direction.
- Get adequate sleep, ideally eight hours per night.
- Talk to your doctor or advanced practice provider about your concerns.

Serena's Story

WE HAVE A PRECIOUS DAUGHTER that we conceived through IVF, and we love her to pieces. We really don't want her to grow up as an only child. My husband and I both carry a problem gene called Fragile X. If the baby inherits the genes, it could result in developmental delay and a whole host of problems. We decided to use one of our remaining embryos that was not affected by the Fragile X abnormal gene from an earlier IVF cycle. We did what is called preimplantation genetic testing to determine whether the embryo is affected. We just had an embryo transfer of a healthy embryo, and luckily I got pregnant. We were delighted when we saw our baby on the ultrasound with its tiny heart beating. Breathtaking! I was doing okay, but at about eight weeks, I started to have spotting and then cramps. I immediately called the doctor. They had me come in and did an ultrasound. The baby died; the doctors called it "embryonic demise." I decided to let nature take its course, and I miscarried on my own. The doctor called me a week later to check in on me. I said I felt fine, but then I started to cry. I lost it. Sobbing, I said, "We don't have any more unaffected embryos, so we now have to do a whole new IVF cycle."

The stress at times feels overwhelming. I do have a good support system with my mom and my husband, who are great. They listen patiently when I cry. I have decided to look at this situation as a cup half-full. We already have a beautiful daughter, and I can do another IVF cycle.

• TAKEAWAY POINTS •

Infertility causes stress. Sometimes, the opposite is true.

Talking with your partner or spouse is a good place to start.

Seek professional care if the stress is affecting your lifestyle.

Acupuncture is an excellent treatment for stress.

A healthy lifestyle is key to obtaining stress relief.

• KEY WORDS •

addressing stress
alternative therapies
silent struggle
stress

REFERENCE

Rooney, K., and A. Domar. 2018. "The Relationship between Stress and Infertility." *Dialogues in Clinical Neuroscience* 20, no. 1, 41–47.

Chapter 20

How to Pay for It All

Financing the Infertility Journey

I'VE BEEN FEELING INDECISIVE and anxious lately. This morning I left agitated for work because my partner, Sha-orong, and I got into an argument about whether to sell his truck. Our arguments have become more frequent lately, as we have been unable to get pregnant for the past two years. At this point our only option is in vitro fertilization (IVF), which can cost $15,000 or more. I've been doing research on the Internet and have looked for loans with low interest, but I also have been thinking about what items I could give up. This is not an easy situation.—*Ying Mei*

What You Need to Know about Paying for Infertility Treatment

The price of infertility treatment varies based on diagnosis and management recommendations of your provider. There is also variability regionally—for example, the price may be lower in South Dakota than it is in New York City. Your health insurance provider may pay for some but not all parts of the infertility evaluation and treatment, making it likely that you will have some out-of-pocket expenses.

Does My Health Care Insurance Cover Infertility Diagnosis and Treatment?

Many health care insurance plans cover diagnostic tests for infertility but not treatment. If you have some options, it would be wise to select a plan that includes infertility treatment. There is significant variability among employers when selecting health care options for employees. Some companies such as Apple, BlackRock, Facebook, and Google cover the cost of egg freezing or embryos and in vitro fertilization. The concept is to encourage women to freeze their eggs when they are younger, allowing them to remain in the workforce. Later, when they are older and decide to start a family, they will have younger, "healthier" eggs available for IVF.

Contact your health care insurance carrier and inquire about coverage for diagnostic tests and for treatment. It is recommended that you work with a financial counselor at the infertility clinic's office, since navigating plan coverage can often be overwhelming. The following states have infertility benefit laws in place:

- Arkansas
- California
- Delaware
- Hawaii
- Illinois
- Louisiana
- Maryland
- Massachusetts
- Montana

- New Hampshire
- New Jersey
- New York
- Ohio
- Rhode Island
- Texas
- Utah
- West Virginia

Once I Decide to Proceed with Treatment, What Might Those Costs Look Like?

When asked about her thoughts regarding financing infertility treatment, one patient aptly stated, "Get a second job and be sure your parents want grandchildren!" Indeed, treatment for infertility can be expensive depending upon what treatments are pursued. Much of the expense for infertility treatment is related to the high cost of medications. If you proceed with **injectable medications** such as for IVF or an injection cycle with medications like Gonal F, Follistim, or Menopur, the costs are high. Pelvic ultrasounds, which are necessary to monitor the ovaries' response to treatment, are also costly. The time that lab personnel spend in preparing a male partner's specimen for insemination or perhaps donor inseminations adds to the cost of the treatment as well. Your health care provider's office should be able to assist you with financing options. Bill coding of tests and procedures is important, and you can inquire about it as the treatment process begins.

Navigating the infertility treatment plan can be taxing on you and your loved ones. Just thinking about the finances can cause stress and anxiety. Luckily, financial counselors at the infertility center can provide excellent advice and options for financing. Their guidance can help minimize the stress related to financing treatment options. Each treatment plan is individualized, so you should discuss your own plan and estimated costs with your doctor's office personnel. No perfect insurance coverage for infertility exists, but because some health care plans cover infertility testing and treatment, you may be able to defray some of the costs.

Approximate Costs by Treatment

Intrauterine Insemination

For some couples, especially in the case of an abnormal semen analysis (male infertility), intrauterine insemination (IUI) may be necessary. IUI may or may not be paired with medications to enhance ovulation. The procedure is done in the office midcycle and involves processing the male sperm specimen to concentrate the sperm most likely to succeed. The sperm are then placed in a syringe and placed through the vagina and cervix directly into the uterus via catheter. The costs vary within a range of $300 to $1,000 for each IUI.

In Vitro Fertilization

IVF cycle costs vary depending upon the amount of medication required to stimulate the ovaries as well as the location of the IVF center. Costs

Average IVF costs, 2023 (varies by region)

IVF cycle	$14,000 or more
Medications	$350 or more
Embryo genetic testing	Varies depending on number of embryos and IVF center
Embryo biopsy	$2,000
Genetics lab charge	Varies by genetics lab
Embryo or egg storage annual fee	$420
Intracytoplasmic sperm injection (ICSI)	$1,600
Assisted hatching of embryo	$540
Anesthesia fee	$1,500
IVF cycle with donor eggs	$38,000

for a new or "fresh" IVF cycle are provided in table 20.1. Some programs have a 100% money back guarantee as part of the treatment plan. These plans are often described as **shared risk plans**.

A number of states mandate that health insurance providers cover IVF:

- Connecticut
- Delaware
- Massachusetts
- New Hampshire
- New Jersey
- New York
- Rhode Island

Some **third-party health care insurance policies** may pay for all or portions of an IVF cycle. It is important to realize that an IVF cycle may not necessarily result in a successful pregnancy. You may need more than one round of IVF.

Egg freezing cycle costs are typically $8,000 to $15,000 based upon the amount of medication required. There is an additional annual fee for storing the eggs.

What Are My Options for Financing?

A number of financing programs are available to help pay for fertility treatment. A few of these are listed below. Some treatment centers provide loans, and a number of infertility practices offer payment plans for certain treatments. You should seek the counsel of a financial counselor to help assess the different packages and options. Some other financing resources are listed on pages 201 and 212.

- RESOLVE: https://www.resolve.org
- Loans for IVF Treatment: http://www.gopher.com
- Lending Club Patient Solutions: https://www.lendingclub.com
- Investopedia: https://www.investopedia.com

In some circumstances, financial assistance is available for IVF, including for teachers and veterans.

What about Financing Fertility Preservation If I Have a Diagnosis of Cancer?

When cancer is diagnosed, a number of grants or scholarships become available to cover IVF or ovarian or sperm tissue freezing. Below are a few of the programs that may help you pursue fertility preservation after a cancer diagnosis.

- Livestrong Fertility Program: https://www.livestrong.org
- Samfund: https://www.allianceforfertilitypreservation.org/the -samfund-scholarship-applications-now-open/
- Gift of Parenthood Grant: https://www.fertilityiq.com

These programs defray all or a significant portion of the cost to freeze eggs, embryos, or ovarian or testicular tissue before cancer therapy, which can have a negative effect on the eggs in the ovaries (or sperm in the testicles).

Janelle's Story

I HAVE BEEN TRYING for the past eight years to have a baby. Today, I celebrated my 45th birthday and realized that my chances of having a baby are getting dimmer with every passing year.

After talking with my doctor, my male partner and I decided that going with donor eggs was our best option. It was a difficult decision because we have limited savings. Even though we both are working, we have to consider the costs of raising a child if we are fortunate enough to have one. We found a great egg bank that gave us lots of good information about potential donors, but we still need to figure out how the heck we were going to pay for this. We searched the Internet for different financial options, such as ARC and Lending Club, after talking to the doctor's office financial counselor. Using RESOLVE's recommendations, we finally decided to use our own personal savings rather than take out a loan. We figured that adding more debt at this point would make us even more financially insecure and stressed. Using our savings, we chose to proceed with an egg bank plan that included a guaranteed blast, which meant that we would be guaranteed to have an embryo to be placed in my uterus. This option was more expensive than the other plans, but at least we will have a chance at being pregnant. After so many years of no success, the guarantee, even though more expensive, gives me a sense that we gave it our best shot. I am apprehensive but hopeful as we begin our journey.

• TAKEAWAY POINTS •

There is no set price to infertility treatment.

Look into your insurance coverage and benefits.

Bill coding of tests and procedures is important.

RESOLVE is a great resource to identify your financial options.

• KEY WORDS •

egg freezing
injectable medications
shared risk plans
third-party health care insurance policies

Chapter 21

The Nontraditional Conception

Donor Insemination, Adopting Embryos, and Beyond

I HAVE GONE THROUGH HELL and back trying to get pregnant. You name the test, and I've had it! They put me on Clomid, had me take shots, suggested IVF cycle after cycle, and nothing. I mean nothing! We have spent a good part of our life savings on this "empty journey." I recently read on a blog about embryo adoption. Intrigued, I thought about exploring this option. Based on what I found, I think this means that I can adopt another couple's embryo and carry it in my uterus. This means I can still carry the pregnancy and give birth. I want to know more!—*Luna*

What You Need to Know about Donor Insemination

If a male has a low sperm count—defined as having fewer than 10 million motile sperm—or if a woman does not have a male partner, donor insemination is a logical approach to conceiving. The process starts with the patient seeking a physician who provides inseminations, usually a reproductive endocrinology infertility specialist. Next is to identify a sperm donor, a process that can often be done online. Most infertility practices have several sperm banks that they recommend, ones that conduct thorough screening and evaluation of donors. Reputable sperm banks obtain detailed medical personal and family histories. Some offer genetic screening of donors. Many sperm banks test the donor for sexually transmitted infections (STIs), and if negative, store the sperm specimens and retest the donor for STIs six months later. Assuming the donor is negative, the specimens are then available for insemination. The bank transports the donor specimens to the infertility center, and the physician then coordinates intrauterine insemination (IUI). The natural cycle or ovulation medications are used to time the insemination. See chapter 3 for further details regarding IUI.

Embryo Adoption

Embryo adoption is an alternative to fertility treatment to have your own biological child. Couples who have undergone in vitro fertilization (IVF) and successfully had a pregnancy may have extra embryos that they do not plan to use. They can elect to let a family interested in adoption undergo embryo transfer of a remaining frozen embryo. The process is similar to adopting a child, only in this case it starts with a donor embryo, and you carry the pregnancy yourself (figure 21.1). One agency that assists with embryo adoptions calls the babies born of embryo adoption "snowflake children." Transferring **ownership** of the embryo from the donor couple to the recipient couple proceeds more or less along the lines of adopting a child.

As time progresses, there are increasingly more embryos available. Some studies estimate there are between 600,000 and 1 million embryos frozen (cryopreserved) in storage. Snowflake embryo adoption agencies are now located across the United States. Embryo adoption, sometimes called embryo donation, has a success rate of over 50%, as reported by a number of snowflake adoption programs.

Egg Banks

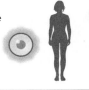

1. Women desiring to donate their eggs go through an IVF cycle
2. Eggs frozen and banked
3. Database of egg donors
4. Selection of donor
5. Eggs shipped to local IVF center for insemination
6. Embryo transfer to recipient

Donor Embryo

1. Couples have completed IVF cycle and have additional frozen embryos
2. Embryos become available for adoption
3. Process somewhat analogous to adopting a child
4. Embryo transferred to local IVF center
5. Embryo transferred to recipient uterus
   who carries the pregnancy

FIGURE 21.1.
Donor egg and embryo options.

Estimating the cost of adopting an embryo is not straightforward and can vary with the agency selected. While one needs to plan to spend in the range of $12,000 to $17,000 for an IVF cycle, in part depending upon the amount of medication required to stimulate the ovaries, the cost for embryo adoption is an average of $8,000 but varies widely.

The **Embryo Awareness Program** was established in 2002 by the US Department of Health and Human Services. On average, the program receives about $1 million in support annually. The grant funds are allocated to select IVF programs and allows select IVF patients to access services that would otherwise not be available to them. Contact these organizations directly to see if you and your partner meet the grant criteria. The umbrella organization for embryo adoption is the National Center for Donor Conception (NCDC). The program also addresses the financial and emotional aspects of the embryo adoption process, which is often complicated. It's not so easy to adopt an embryo.

Embryo adoption can be an alternative for nontraditional family building, including LGBTQ+ parents, as well as single individuals pursuing parenthood. Agencies vary with respect to donor and recipient candidates.

What You Need to Know about Adopting a Child

Another route to parenthood is to adopt a baby. Cost must be considered, as your budget may determine what options are available to you. As an estimate, costs ranging from $20,000 to $30,000 can be expected.

There are many domestic and international adoption programs and agencies to help you adopt a child. One good source for information is the **Adoption Network**. The criteria for adoption will differ depending on whether you wish to adopt an infant as opposed to an older child. Private adoption agencies and foster care programs exist, as well as open, semi-open, and closed adoption options.

The process of adopting a child can be challenging to say the least. Here are some questions to ask any agency you are considering to help you navigate the process:

1. What type of children does the agency place (age and background)?
2. How does the agency identify children for adoption, and what information is obtained regarding the parent(s) giving up the child for adoption?
3. What is the estimated timeline?
4. What information about me (home study) does the agency collect?
5. Does the home study involve social services?
6. What is the cost?
7. What are the options for financial protection if the adoption falls through?
8. Are adoption professionals available to help with:
   a. creating an adoption plan?
   b. creating an adoption parent profile?
9. How is official approval for the adoption obtained?

10. At what point can I view a list of older children available for adoption?
11. If I have chosen to adopt a newborn, do adoptive parents have the option to move forward or decline the opportunity?

There are many legal aspects to consider with regard to adopting an unborn child. Once the child is placed, a postadoption supervisory assessment and report occurs. Details of this assessment include how the new parents are adjusting to the child, along with the child's developmental milestones and activities of daily living. There may also be an evaluation of the physical alterations in the home, finances, and age-appropriate child schedules. Once the child has bonded with the adoptive parents, and the birth parents are comfortable with the arrangement, the adoption can be finalized legally.

The Internet is a good source of information on adoption. The following sites can help you navigate the ins and outs of the process.

- www.adoptionnetwork.com
- www.adoptionstar.com
- www.adopt.org
- www.adoptivefamilies.com
- www.americanadoptions.com
- www.nacac.org
- www.nolo.com
- www.nonprofitquarterly.org
- www.ocfs.ny.gov
- www.travel.state.gov

Gestational Carrier and Surrogacy

The practice of using gestational carrier or a gestational surrogate is common around the globe. There are various legal and ethical implications of using gestational carriers.

It is important to define the language surrounding this practice, as different phrases carry different meanings depending on the situation. A gestational carrier (sometimes called a "surrogate," although "gestational carrier" is often the preferred term) is defined as a person who agrees to have an embryo implanted into her uterus, with plans to carry that pregnancy and deliver for the intended parents, who are unable to conceive for whatever reason.

A "traditional surrogate" or "straight surrogate" is when a woman undergoes artificial insemination with the intended parent's sperm, thus using both her eggs and uterus to carry the pregnancy. Traditional or straight surrogates have a genetic relationship to the pregnancy. This practice is widely deemed as unethical and rarely practiced.

Commercial surrogacy is when a person serves as a gestational carrier for payment. The surrogate is compensated for carrying the pregnancy and is reimbursed for all medical costs. Altruistic surrogacy is when a person serves as a gestational carrier without payment, and only receives reimbursement for medical costs.

The intended parents are the couple or individual who intends to parent the delivered child/children from the pregnancy carried by a gestational carrier.

The practice of gestational surrogacy within the United States and around the globe has many different legal implications. Commercial surrogacy, where payment along with reimbursement for medical costs is made to the surrogate, is legal in the countries of Georgia, Israel, Russia, Thailand, Ukraine, and the United States. In the United States, there is no federal law legalizing commercial surrogacy; only at the state level are there laws pertaining to commercial surrogacy. In Thailand, commercial surrogacy is legal only for heterosexual couples.

In Australia, Belgium, Canada, the Czech Republic, Denmark, Greece, Holland, India, New Zealand, Portugal, South Africa, and the United Kingdom, only altruistic surrogacy is legal; commercial gestational surrogacy is illegal. In India, only heterosexuals are allowed to pursue altruistic gestational surrogacy.

Some countries outlaw all forms of gestational carrying and gestational surrogacy: Brazil, France, Germany, Ireland, Italy, Lithuania, and Spain. Surrogacy is also illegal in China, but it is still very common and frequently practiced. There are known to be 300 to 500 infertility clinics across the country.

The practice of gestational carrying has important ethical considerations as well. In India, gestational carrying was legal from 2002 to 2018. This resulted in a $2.6 billion industry annually. With the massive profit from the practice, many young women were placed in vulnerable situations as surrogacy quickly became less and less regulated. In 2018, the practice of gestational carrying was deemed illegal, and now altruistic surrogacy is the only type of gestational surrogacy allowed.

Surrogacy has led to dangerous ties to human trafficking across the globe. In Nigeria, despite the fact that the practice is illegal, there are well-known "baby factories," which are large, abandoned houses or buildings that house young women who are carrying pregnancies for people from outside countries. Once born, these babies are sold into human trafficking. The unregulated practice of gestational carrying can lead to horrific outcomes.

Within the United States, the practice of gestational carrying is highly regulated. Between 1999 and 2013, there were 30,927 pregnancies from gestational surrogacy. The practice has additionally been on the rise. In 2015, 750 pregnancies were born from gestational carriers. In 2021, 2,800 pregnancies were from gestational carriers.

There are specific legal terms regarding gestational carrying in the United States. A pre-birth order is an agreement signed by the gestational carrier, the intended parents, and a judge that declares the legal parentage of the baby to be born. A post-birth order is an agreement signed by the gestational carrier, intended parents, and a judge that declares the legal parentage of the baby only after it is born.

There are no current federal regulations surrounding gestational carrying in the United States. All laws are at the state level. Commercial surrogacy is illegal in Louisiana, Michigan, and Nebraska.

It is more difficult in some states than others for the intended parents to obtain a pre-birth or post-birth order. In California, pre-birth orders are granted for intended parents whether they are married, unmarried, heterosexual, homosexual, or single parents. Other states grant pre-birth orders only in specific situations, such as for married couples or parents who have a genetic relationship to the baby born, meaning that there can be no use of egg or sperm donors. In Idaho and Wyoming, only post-birth orders are granted.

It is very important for families to explore legal counsel early on if they hope to utilize a gestational carrier, since the laws vary greatly from state to state.

Gianna's Story

I KNEW AS SOON AS WE TOOK her home that she would be a very special baby. We were so frustrated when the first adoption fell through at the last minute. The mom decided to keep the baby once she heard her cry in the delivery room. We had everything ready—the room was painted, the crib assembled. We were incredibly excited, and then the phone call from our attorney came: "The mother decided to keep the baby." Need I say more how depressing it turned out to be. But we remained hopeful. The second time around, it all came together. She is absolutely incredible, and my heart is full as I hold her in my arms.

• TAKEAWAY POINTS •

Embryo adoption agencies are available worldwide.

Adopting a baby or a child requires preliminary evaluation.

Adoption agencies facilitate the process.

Do your research on the process so that you are prepared.

• KEY WORDS •

Adoption Network
embryo adoption
Embryo Awareness Program
ownership

REFERENCE

Lester, Caroline. 2019. "Embryo 'Adoption' Is Growing, but It's Getting Tangled in the Abortion Debate." *New York Times*, February 17, 2019. https://www.nytimes.com/2019/02/17/health/embryo-adoption-donated-snowflake.html

Chapter 22

The End Is in Sight

You're Pregnant—What's Next?

I'M DISCOURAGED. We have been trying to get pregnant for over three years. My husband is great—my true soul mate—and always cheers me up. But then again, six Clomid cycles with IUI (intrauterine insemination) and no luck for us. After these trials we decided to proceed with IVF (in vitro fertilization). We did test after test. We talked with the financial counselor and picked the best plan that had a "money back guarantee."

Now is the waiting game to see if I get my period. One week, two weeks, and nothing. No cramps, my breasts are tender, and I am peeing a lot. I went to the pharmacy and got a home pregnancy test. I peed on the stick, and it was positive! Not convinced of the results, I went out and got a different pregnancy test. Again it was positive. I called my doctor and scheduled a blood pregnancy test, which showed a good number. We followed up with an ultrasound, and so far the pregnancy is going well.

Can this be the answer to my prayers?—*Mera*

What You Need to Know Once You're Pregnant

Disclosure: The following information includes general recommendations for do's and don'ts during pregnancy; however, further updated reports and research may alter these guidelines. Please reach out to your OB-GYN or other health provider to ensure that you have the most up-to-date information.

Once you are late for a period, a urine pregnancy test is usually the first step in determining a pregnancy. Your health care provider may do a blood test to determine your HCG (human chorionic gonadotropin) value. Sometimes the progress and status of the pregnancy are monitored by repeating the blood pregnancy test to determine whether the value is appropriately rising. An appropriate rise would indicate a normal pregnancy. Your provider may obtain an ultrasound to confirm that the pregnancy is in the uterus and ultimately has a heartbeat (at six weeks or later).

Let's talk about **nutrition** in pregnancy. A well-balanced diet that includes adequate protein (the building blocks of life) complemented by appropriate amounts of carbohydrate and "good" fats sets the stage for fetal development. **Omega fatty acids** including DHA (docosahexaenoic acid) are beneficial. Omega-3 fatty acids are better than omega-6 fatty acids. Choline and fat-soluble nutrients are also good for you; fish, grass-fed meat, and pasture-raised eggs are good sources. Vitamin and mineral supplements, including prenatal vitamins, are important. Be sure to discuss with your health care provider the minimum daily requirements of **vitamins** and **minerals**, especially vitamins A, D, and E. Also critical are the B complex vitamins, including B_{12}, and vitamin K complemented by iron, calcium, and magnesium. By following these nutritional guidelines, you set the stage for good fetal growth and development.

What Foods Should I Avoid?

It is a good idea to avoid refined sugars when you are pregnant or trying to get pregnant. The following have high sugar contents:

- Whole sugar
- Brown sugar
- Raw sugar
- Molasses
- Honey
- Corn syrup
- Soda
- Punch
- Barbeque sauce
- Ketchup

You should also avoid artificial sweeteners, although steviosides (and other sweeteners derived from stevia) and erythritol are okay if you are looking for sweetness without the sugar. The following artificial sweeteners are not good choices, however, and should be avoided:

- Aspartame
- Sucralose
- Saccharine
- Acesulfame potassium
- Neotame

While you are pregnant, it is best to avoid eating sushi, hot dogs, deli-cut meats, and unpasteurized cheeses. Meats sliced in a deli can harbor bacteria. Spicy foods may cause indigestion more easily during pregnancy, as the hormones affect your stomach and gastrointestinal tract.

Regarding fish, you should avoid or minimize your consumption of "bottom feeders" that are high in mercury:

- Bigeye tuna
- Tilefish
- Shark
- Swordfish
- Marlin

- Orange roughy
- King mackerel

Most canned tuna is okay during pregnancy, as recommended by the American College of Obstetricians and Gynecologists.

What about Smoking and Drinking?

Smoking is bad for your health whether you are pregnant or not. You should also try to avoid secondhand smoke from the people around you.

Do not drink alcohol during pregnancy, as there is no safe amount of alcohol for a developing fetus. If you find you are having trouble stopping drinking, you should reach out to your health care provider for help.

Should I Be Worried about Morning Sickness?

Morning sickness is not uncommon and is caused by the pregnancy hormones. If you are experiencing morning sickness, try eating light meals throughout the course of the day instead of three large meals. Taking 200 milligrams of **ginger** (ginger ale is inadequate) every six hours may also help. It may also help to suck on hard lozenges (some brands are made specifically for morning sickness) when you are feeling nauseated.

If your nausea does not improve or if you are having trouble keeping food down, you may have a more serious form of morning sickness called "hyperemesis gravidarum." Consult with your doctor if you are concerned about your morning sickness.

How Much Should I Exercise?

It is safe to exercise in moderation while you are pregnant. Discuss your level of activity and specific exercise program with your health care provider. In general, high-impact sports, any activity with the potential for a hard fall such as downhill skiing, scuba diving, and heavy lifting are best avoided during pregnancy.

How Long Should I Wait between Pregnancies?

The American College of Obstetricans and Gynecologists consensus opinion recommends at least a six-month interval between pregnancies. In general, providers recommend up to at least 18 months between giving birth and your next pregnancy.

Xia's Story

SHE'S BEAUTIFUL! We waited a long time for her to arrive—we tried to get pregnant for four years—but that's history. She was worth every step of the effort!

The doctor put me on Clomid pills by mouth for five days. I checked for ovulation and told them if I had a color change on my ovulation predictor kit. Part of the process was I had to take one shot to release my egg, and we had to have sex right around that time. They called this "timed intercourse." I then went on the vaginal progesterone every day. For the first three months of my pregnancy, I had to take vaginal natural progesterone tablets.

The pregnancy went well, but I did experience nausea for the first three months. My labor lasted three hours, and I had to push for about 45 minutes. We could see her head coming out; she had lots of dark hair, just like my husband. She started to cry immediately, and as I held her, I could not stop my tears of joy. Yeah, she cries at night—usually it's because she is hungry. I'm breastfeeding and love the opportunity to hold her so close to me.

• TAKEAWAY POINTS •

Good nutrition is critical for a healthy pregnancy, both for mom and baby.

Certain foods should be avoided.

Do not smoke, and avoid secondhand smoke.

Do not drink alcohol while you are pregnant.

A moderate exercise program that has a low risk of falls is best during pregnancy.

Ginger can help with morning sickness.

• KEY WORDS •

ginger
minerals
nutrition
omega fatty acids
pregnancy interval
vitamins

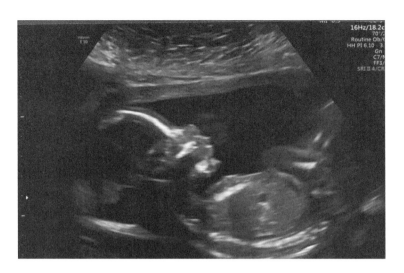

Ultrasound at 4.5 months.

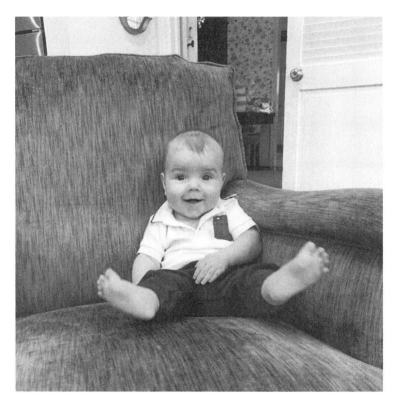

Remember: miracles take time.

Final Words

One's plans to get pregnant, have a baby, and live happily ever after are often interrupted by infertility. Globally, 48.5 million couples experience infertility, representing 15% of all couples. About 9% of men and 10% of women aged 15 to 44 reported infertility problems in the United States (Centers for Disease Control and Prevention, 2022; Office on Women's Health, 2022).

As the personal stories in this book attest, infertility can be anxiety-provoking, stressful, and at times depressing. But there is light at the end of the tunnel, as there are multiple ways to become a parent and build a family. Understanding what an individual or couple has gone through can help provide you with a sense of what to expect or ease your concerns about the trials and tribulations of infertility.

The information we provide is designed to assist you in timing intercourse with ovulation, understanding the multiple facets of infertility, and communicating with your doctor. We have suggested apps to facilitate you with identifying ovulation. We've also described how lifestyle, diet, exercise, and other factors can help improve your natural fertility. Giving couples much-needed information on what they can do to improve their fertility is one of the main goals of this book.

We have presented the multiple components of female infertility, such as endometriosis, uterine fibroids, ovarian reserve (egg supply), and tubal factors, in a readily understandable format. Female problems such as abnormal menstrual cycles, pelvic pain, endometriosis, and uterine fibroids are medical challenges that intertwine with infertility. Advances in both the science and the art of medicine have brought many new treatment options for such conditions.

We also have covered male factors accounting for inability to conceive, including erectile dysfunction and low sperm counts, as well as the reasons these problems may occur. The state of knowledge regarding male infertility continues to improve. More recent research focuses on sperm DNA fragmentation, providing additional information about sperm DNA and sperm's ability to penetrate the oocyte, resulting in fertilization. For more information on this topic, see Agarwal et al. (2020).

A link exists between recurrent miscarriages and reproductive immunology. Sometimes the uterus will "reject" proper embryo implantation. Treatment can include but is not limited to anticoagulants. A beautiful baby may still be the result. The terminology we use, "to viability," meaning perhaps you didn't go a full nine months but progressed to such a degree that the baby survives, is an important term to know. This outcome may include time for the baby in a neonatal intensive care unit (NICU).

The topic of sexual dysfunction is a challenge to say the least. Men may feel frustration about "having to have sex" during ovulation. The pressure can result in erectile dysfunction. Decreasing libido among couples experiencing infertility is a problem we clinicians face with increasing frequency. Getting to the root cause and emphasizing the importance of communication and support between the couple can be challenging for the practitioner, physician, or advanced practice provider. Psychologists and sex therapists certified by the American Association of Sexuality Educators, Counselors and Therapists (AASECT) who are experienced in sexual dysfunction can be instrumental in caring for infertile couples. For sexual dysfunction that persists, new medications and devices are helping couples become pregnant. Intrauterine inseminations can be of assistance depending upon the sperm count.

188 • The Expert Guide to Fertility

The advent of in vitro fertilization with ICSI (intracytoplasmic sperm injection) has allowed many men with abnormal sperm counts to have their own biological child.

New advances in the treatment of recurrent miscarriages are helping more women carry a baby to term (nine months). In vitro fertilization with preimplantation genetic embryo testing can identify genetically normal embryos, improving the chance of successful implantation and progression on to a healthy baby.

In vitro fertilization is now a technical advance that spans over 45 years and is responsible for more than 10 million babies worldwide. In one sense none of these babies—individuals—would be here today without the expertise of many researchers and clinicians. The tradition of IVF continues to reach new horizons.

We need to recognize our military and take a moment to thank each and every service member for their willingness to defend our country and allow us to continue to be the most well-respected nation in the world. Military benefits now cover some infertility services, facilitating the process of becoming a parent that our men and women in uniform are so deserving of.

Today there is greater acceptance of and support for nontraditional families than ever before. Lesbian, gay, bisexual, transgender, and queer (LGBTQ) couples now have at their disposal a whole gamut of fertility treatment options for conception, pregnancy, and the future.

Advances in cancer treatment have resulted in not only "life after cancer," but also ever-enhanced quality of life. Preservation of eggs, sperm, and ovarian or testicular tissue prior to chemo or radiation therapy allows an individual to have their own biological, genetic child. Reproductive endocrine infertility specialists continue to work well with oncologists to preserve fertility before cancer treatment begins.

So many topics, such as stress related to infertility, donor inseminations, and embryo adoption, need to be better understood and facilitated. Access to this information is in part a significant objective of the book. We hope we have opened the door for many of you to learn about the options and future directions of infertility treatment.

Don't lose hope, keep a positive attitude, and remember that we the physicians, advanced practice providers, nurses, and office staff are here to assist you. We too learn from our patients as we progress. The journey at times is challenging, but support is readily available.

Wishing you every success. Best to you.

Joseph S. Sanfilippo, MD, MBA
Aarti Kumar, MD

REFERENCES

Agarwal, Ashok, Ahmad Majzoub, Saradha Baskaran, Manesh Kumar Panner Selvam, Chak Lam Cho, et al. 2020. "Sperm DNA Fragmentation: A New Guideline for Clinicians." *World Journal of Men's Health* 38, no. 4: 412–71. doi:10.5534/wjmh.200128

Centers for Disease Control and Prevention. 2022. "Women's Health." Last updated September 29, 2022. https://www.cdc.gov/women/index.htm

Office on Women's Health. 2022. "Infertility." Accessed December 16, 2022. https://www.womenshealth.gov/a-z-topics/infertility

Acknowledgments

CLW has been incredibly valuable in providing you, the reader, with "the patient's perspective." She has shared her trials and tribulations along the path toward fertility, which ultimately was successful. Her input in almost every chapter provides a unique look at "what it's really like"—what has worked, what has been stressful, and suggestions on how to cope at various points along the challenging journey. We are all indebted to her for her candor and guidance to help you have success with the challenge of infertility.

Caitlin Lazzaro, RN, has expertise in infertility. She comes to us from the nursing perspective as part of the health care team. This cohort includes physicians, advanced practice providers, nurses, IVF lab personnel, and administrative staff. She is a most reliable resource and advocate for patients. We are grateful to her for her dedication and expertise.

Susan Dunlow, MD, is an OB-GYN dedicated to educating students, residents, and attending physicians. With a career dedicated to "military medicine," Dr. Dunlow has shared her expertise regarding the challenges military personnel face when pursuing infertility treatment. We hope the information proves useful for our heroic military members who are navigating infertility evaluation and treatment.

Natalie Nakles, MD, has shared her talents by contributing to the illustrations in this book. Dr. Nakles is a most gifted physician-artist with a keen understanding of anatomy and physiology. We are grateful for her expertise and contributions to our book.

Dr. Rita Kumar, executive director of the Faculty Enrichment Center at the University of Cincinnati, is a dedicated professor of English. She has been extremely patient with the process of editing our book, sharing her command of the English language and excellent communication skills. Her ability to provide succinct and targeted information facilitates you, the reader, in understanding all the details provided throughout the book.

John Silpigni, director of Health Case Management (Social Service) at Magee-Women's Hospital, has provided direction and expertise with regard to the social services aspects of infertility patient care. Mr. Silpigni has been a tremendous asset to this book.

Carlie Magner, PA-C, has been helpful in identifying specific patients who were willing to share their experience with infertility. An advanced practice provider, Carlie is a true patient advocate and is most competent regarding infertility patient care.

Roshni Ray, MD, as a medical student from University of Texas, San Antonio, shared her knowledge and understanding of infertility patient care. With a focus on underserved patient populations, she provided tireless hours of input, chapter by chapter. It has been most appreciated.

L.L. is a patient who has willingly shared her experience, frustration, excitement, and joy. She provided us with an education from the perspective of going through infertility as part of a same-sex couple and the specific barriers that needed to be addressed. We are most grateful and hope her successful experience proves beneficial to our readers.

Joan Parker, president of Parker Literary Agency, LLC, has been most valuable in assisting us with details of the publishing process and preparation of our book. We thank her for her expertise.

Kathleen Gustafson, imaging services supervisor, and Lanita Johnson, sonographer, were instrumental in assisting with ultrasound images.

Caroline Ayinon, MD, assisted with the illustrations in this book.

Caroline Kettering, MD, helped us with manuscript preparation.

Meghan Schneck, PA-C, shared information regarding social media and what is particularly pertinent to infertility patients. Her knowledge and expertise are greatly appreciated.

Hannah Shepard, PA-C, assisted with specific aspects of social media.

Thanks to physician assistant K.P. for her constructive input and assistance with illustrations.

Thanks to Megan Kukic Rozewicz, RN, for her assistance with organization of the book and suggested chapter titles.

Thanks to S. and R.L. for their willingness to share their ultrasound image.

Jane Whitney is appreciated for her talent and expertise in the provision of illustrations.

Will Holmes provided constructive input on text throughout the book.

Joseph Rusko, editor at Johns Hopkins University Press, offered constructive input and assistance.

We hope the input, experience, and expertise of these individuals have assisted you in your journey through infertility.

The patience and knowledge of nursing staff all over the world have been indispensable to infertility patients. We thank them for their time and dedication.

Advanced practice practitioners that we have worked with, both physician assistants and nurse practitioners, are to be recognized for their expertise. These individuals are extremely well versed with infertility evaluation and management. They have been and continue to be leaders in providing care for infertility patients. Thank you!

Resources

Overview

You will see the following organizations show up in a majority of the chapter resources: the American College of Obstetricians and Gynecologists (ACOG), the American Academy of Family Physicians (AAFP), the American Society of Reproductive Medicine (ASRM), and RESOLVE, which is also known as the National Infertility Association. For each chapter, we recommend certain search topics relevant to the chapter that can be found on the home websites of these organizations:

ACOG: acog.org
AAFP: aafp.org
ASRM: asrm.org
RESOLVE: resolve.org

One excellent resource to explore your options is the National Infertility Association. Their website, resolve.org, lists a number of support groups throughout the United States and can answer questions about insurance coverage, psychological support, and a number of other related topics.

Note: These resources only scratch the surface of the available information about women's health, pregnancy, and infertility. Many of the podcasts and YouTube channels touch on more topics than what is listed here. Feel free to dig deeper into these platforms to find the right episodes and content for you.

Disclaimer: We cannot vouch for the validity of nor assume responsibility for any potential adverse consequences of content shared on social media.

Chapter 2. Enhancing Your Chances: Optimizing Natural Fertility

American Academy of Family Physicians: www.aafp.org
   Preconception Counseling
American College of Obstetricians and Gynecologists: www.acog.org
   Prepregnancy Counseling
American Society for Reproductive Medicine: www.asrm.org
   Optimizing Natural Fertility

American Pregnancy Association: www.americanpregnancy.org

Centers for Disease Control and Prevention. 2022. "Before Pregnancy." Last reviewed September 20, 2022. https://www.cdc.gov/preconception/index.html

March of Dimes. 2020. "Getting Ready for Pregnancy: Preconception Health." Last reviewed September 2020. https://www.marchofdimes.org/pregnancy /getting-ready-for-pregnancy-preconception-health.aspx

National Preconception Health and Health Care Initiative. 2014. *Before, Between, and Beyond Pregnancy: The National Preconception Curriculum and Resources Guide for Clinicians*. Chapel Hill, NC: National Preconception Health and Health Care Initiative.

Chapter 3. *Against All Odds: Female Infertility*

American Academy of Family Physicians: www.aafp.org
Evaluation and Treatment of Infertility

American College of Obstetricians and Gynecologists: www.acog.org
Treating Infertility

American Society for Reproductive Medicine: www.asrm.org
Infertility

RESOLVE, The National Infertility Association: www.resolve.org

Chapter 4. *We're Part of It, Too: Male Infertility*

American Society for Reproductive Medicine: www.asrm.org
Diagnosis and Treatment of Infertility in Men

American Urology Association: http://www.auanet.org/guidelines-and-quality /guidelines/male-infertility

Male infertility and sexual dysfunction: www.malefertility.com

RESOLVE, The National Infertility Association: www.resolve.org
Male Factor Infertility

UpToDate: http://www.auanet.org/guidelines-and-quality/guidelines/male-infertility

Chapter 5. *The Embryo Just Won't Stick: Reproductive Immunology*

Alan E. Beer Medical Center for Reproductive Immunology: www.repro-med.net
American Society for Reproductive Immunology: www.theasri.org
CNY Fertility: www.cnyfertility.com/inflammation-and-reproductive-immunology/
International Federation of Fertility Societies (IFFS): www.iffsreproduction.org
International Society for In Vitro Fertilization: www.isivf.com

National Institute of Child Health and Human Development, Reproductive
Sciences Branch: www.nichd.nih.gov

Reproductive immunology support resources: www.immunologysupport.com

Chapter 6. Not Tonight, Wait till Ovulation: Sexual Dysfunction

American Association of Couples and Sex Therapists: www.aacast.net

American Association of Sexuality Educators: www.assect.org

American College of Obstetricians and Gynecologists. 2019. "Female Sexual
Dysfunction: ACOG Practice Bulletin Clinical Management Guidelines for
Obstetrician-Gynecologists, Number 213." *Obstetrics and Gynecology* 134: e1–18.

American Psychiatric Association. 2013. *Diagnostic and Statistical Manual of Mental
Disorders*, 5th ed. Washington, DC: American Psychiatric Association.

American Psychological Association: www.apa.org/topics/sex-sexuality/treatment

Boston Medical Group: www.bostonmedicalgroup.com/the-boston-method
/treatment-options/

International Society for Sexual Medicine: www.issm.info

Kingsberg, S., et al. 2017. "Female Sexual Dysfunction—Medical and Psychological
Treatments." *Journal of Sexual Medicine* 14, no. 12: 1463–91.

"Pioneering 'Masters of Sex' Brought Science to the Bedroom." NPR, October 4,
2013. https://www.npr.org/2013/10/04/228906644/pioneering-masters-of
-sex-brought-science-to-the-bedroom.

Society for Sex Therapy and Research: www.sstarnet.org

Chapter 7. No Periods for Me: Amenorrhea

For more information, enter the search term "Amenorrhea" on any of the following
websites.

American Academy of Family Practice: www.aafp.org

American College of Obstetricians and Gynecologists: www.acog.org

American Society for Reproductive Medicine: www.asrm.org

Chapter 8. I Just Can't Stop Bleeding: Abnormal Vaginal Bleeding

For more information, enter the search term "Abnormal Uterine Bleeding" on any
of the following websites.

American Academy of Family Practice: www.aafp.org

American College of Obstetricians and Gynecologists: www.acog.org

American Society for Reproductive Medicine: www.asrm.org

Chapter 9. Painful Periods, Nobody's Listening: Endometriosis

American College of Obstetricians and Gynecologists: www.acog.org
Endometriosis
American Society for Reproductive Medicine: www.asrm.org
Endometriosis
Endometriosis Association: www.endometriosisassn.org
Endometriosis Support Group: www.myendometriosisteam.com

Chapter 10. I Have Acne, I'm Hairy, and I Just Can't Get Pregnant: Polycystic Ovaries

American Association of Family Practice: www.aafp.org
PCOS
American College of Obstetricians and Gynecologists: www.acog.org
PCOS
American Society for Reproductive Medicine: www.asrm.org
PCOS
Androgen Excess Society: www.ae-society.org
PCOS Awareness Association: www.pcosaa.org
PCOS Foundation: www.pcosfoundation.org

Chapter 11. No Room for the Fetus: Uterine Fibroids

American Association of Family Practice: www.aafp.org
Uterine Fibroids
American College of Obstetricians and Gynecologists: www.acog.org
Uterine Fibroids
American Society for Reproductive Medicine: www.asrm.org
Fibroids or Myomas
Fibroid Centers: www.usafibroidcenters.com

Chapter 12. Too Little, Too Early: Miscarriages

American College of Obstetricians and Gynecologists: www.acog.org
Early Pregnancy Loss
American Psychological Association: www.apa.org
Miscarriage and Loss

American Society for Reproductive Medicine: www.asrm.org
  Miscarriage or Recurrent Pregnancy Loss
Hohn, Ingrid, and Perry-Lynn Moffet. 1992. *A Silent Sorrow: Pregnancy Loss*. New
  York: Dell.
March of Dimes: www.marchofdimes.org
  Miscarriage, Loss, and Grief
Pregnancy Loss Support Program: www.pregnancyloss.org

Chapter 13. Wrong Place, Painful Conception: Ectopic Pregnancy

American Academy of Family Physicians: www.aafp.org
  Diagnosis and Management of Ectopic Pregnancy
American College of Obstetricians and Gynecologists: www.acog.org
  Ectopic Pregnancy
Reproductive Facts: www.reproductivefacts.org

Chapter 14. Help Is Here: Assisted Reproductive Technology

American Society for Reproductive Endocrinology: www.asrm.org
  Assisted Reproductive Technology
International Federation of Fertility Societies: www.iffsreproduction.org
International Society for In Vitro Fertilization: www.isivf.com
RESOLVE: The National Infertility Association: www.resolve.org
  Assisted Reproductive Technology Myths and Facts
Society for Assisted Reproductive Technology: www.sart.org

Chapter 15. Keep My Eggs Ripe: Social Egg Freezing

American Society for Reproductive Endocrinology: www.asrm.org
  Cryopreservation and Storage
Progny: Fertility Benefits Management Company, Progny.com
Society for Assisted Reproductive Technology: www.sart.org
TMRW Life Sciences: www.tmrw.org

Chapter 16. Cancer Can't Stop Me: Fertility Preservation

American Academy of Pediatrics: www.aap.org
  Fertility Preservation for Pediatric and Adolescent Patients with
  Cancer

American Cancer Society: www.cancer.org
   Female Fertility and Cancer
American Society of Clinical Oncology: www.asco.org
   Fertility Preservation in Patients with Cancer
American Society for Reproductive Medicine: www.asrm.org
   Fertility Preservation in Female Cancer Patients

Chapter 17. Building a Nontraditional Family: Nonbinary Fertility

American College of Obstetricians and Gynecologists: www.acog.org
   Marriage and Family Building Equality
American Society for Reproductive Medicine: www.asrm.org
   LGBTQ+ Family Building through ART
Family Equality: www.familyequality.org
Gay Parents Magazine: gayparentmag.com
Nahata, Leena, Lisa T. Campo-Engelstein, Amy Tishelman, Gwendolyn P. Quinn,
   and John D. Lantos. 2018. "Fertility Preservation for a Transgender Teenager."
   Pediatrics 142, no. 3: e20173142. https://doi.org/10.1542/peds.2017-3142
RESOLVE, The National Infertility Association: www.resolve.org
   LGBTQ+ family building options
World Professional Association for Transgender Health: www.wpath.org

Chapter 18. Building a Family While Serving the Nation: Military Fertility Services

Kerslake, Risa. 2021. "Infertility Presents Unique Challenges for Military
   Families." *Military Families*, April 27, 2021. https://militaryfamilies.com
   /military-health/infertility-presents-unique-challenges-for-military-families/
RESOLVE, The National Fertility Association: www.resolve.org
   Military Personnel Options
TRICARE: www.tricare.mil
   Fertility Insurance Benefits

Chapter 19. Help Me Preserve My Sanity: Managing Stress

See the multiple patient experience YouTube videos, podcasts, and media references
   below for additional resources.
Assisted Reproductive Services: www.tricare.mil/CoveredServices/IsItCovered/
   AssistedReproductiveServices

Circle and Bloom: www.circlebloom.com

Emotional Freedom Technique: www.goodtherapy.org/learn-about-therapy/types
/emotional-freedom-technique

Fertility Rally: www.fertilityrally.com

Reproductive Health Care Coverage: www.tricare.mil/CoveredServices/
Reproductive-Health

RESOLVE, The National Infertility Association: www.resolve.org
Managing Infertility Stress

Reproductivefacts.org
Stress and Infertility, Patient Video

Rooney, Kristin L. 2018. "The Relationship between Stress and Infertility."
Dialogues in Clinical Neuroscience 20, no. 1: 41–47. doi:10.31887/DCNS.2018.20.1/
klrooney

Chapter 20. How to Pay for It All: Financing the Infertility Journey

RESOLVE (www.resolve.org) provides information about the following finance
topics, among others.

Getting Insurance Coverage	Financing Adoptions
Making Infertility Affordable	Financial Relief for Infertility
Medication Discounts	Infertility Treatment Grants

Many other financial resources exist to help you pay for infertility treatment. Below
are some options you may find helpful.

ARC Fertility: www.arcfertility.com

- ARC Cycle Plus Program: egg retrieval and up to two embryo transfers
- ARC Egg Donor Packages and LGBTQ Family-Building Programs
- ARC Egg Freezing Package
- ARC Success Program: discounted multicycle program with a refund on
unused cycles

Family Equality: www.familyequality.org

Chapter 21. The Nontraditional Conception: Donor Insemination, Adopting Embryos, and Beyond

American Embryo Adoption Agency: www.embryoadoptionusa.com

American Society for Reproductive Medicine: www.asrm.org
Guidance Regarding Gamete and Embryo Donation
Insemination

Sperm Donation

Third-Party Reproduction

Donor Conception Network: www.dcnetwork.org

National Embryo Donation Center: www.embryodonation.org

RESOLVE, The National Infertility Association: www.resolve.org

Donor Options

Chapter 22. The End Is in Sight: You're Pregnant—What's Next?

Baby Center: www.babycenter.com

This resource will help you learn about each milestone in pregnancy.

Early Childhood Learning and Knowledge Center: www.eclkc.ohs.acf.hhs.gov

Mother to Baby: www.mothertobaby.org

Parenting 24/7: www.parenting247.org

24 Websites Every Pregnant Woman Should Know About: www.mothersniche.com

US Breastfeeding Committee: www.usbreastfeeding.org

Work and Life Balance: www.familiesandwork.org

Social Media, Podcasts, Apps, and More

Infertility

Social Media

Facebook: TTC, Infertility, Pregnancy Support Group

Public support group run by multiple women who have previously experienced or are currently experiencing infertility. This group has 50+ posts daily. TTC stands for "trying to conceive."

Podcasts

Fertility Docs Uncensored

Hosts Brandy Thomas, Carrie Bedient, MD, Susan Hudson, MD, and Abby Eblen, MD, debunk the myths and echo the truths regarding common misconceptions of infertility.

As a Woman

Host Natalie Crawford, MD, is a board-certified physician in both obstetrics and gynecology as well as reproductive endocrinology and infertility who has thoughtfully crafted a podcast to educate and empower women who struggle with infertility.

Infertile AF

Alison Prato, a journalist located in Brooklyn, New York, shares touching, true stories from both men and women who are undergoing the infertility journey. Each weekly episode reveals a new story.

Fab Fertility

Host Blair Nelson provides all the necessary details regarding infertility treatment, IVF, her personal battles, and more.

The OB/GYN Podcast: Season 1, Episode 69, "Infertility Work-Up"

Led by Dr. Joseph Chappelle and frequented by guest speakers, this podcast goes the extra mile for the science minded. *The OB/GYN Podcast* provides comprehensive explanations of the most pertinent topics in the field. The above episode, hosted by Jillian Kurtz, DO, is an in-depth, 17-minute discussion of the steps included in an infertility workup.

The Skinny Confidential Him and Her Podcast: Episodes 344 and 404

Husband-and-wife duo Michael Bosstick and Lauryn Evarts ask the questions that may be on your mind about infertility, egg freezing, embryo transfer, and more. Although infertility is an undoubtedly heavy and serious topic, the couple provides a lighter approach and makes the listener feel engaged and part of the conversation. We recommend Episodes 344 and 404, in which the hosts interview expert Shahin Ghadir, MD.

The Fertile Life

Fertility expert Dr. Shahin Ghadir interviews guests about their paths to parenthood and dives into discussions about how becoming a parent differs for all. The hope of this podcast is to create a guide for listeners in all stages of life, as well as break the stigmas often associated with fertility.

Apps

Clue

Clue is a comprehensive menstrual cycle and ovulation calendar app that includes symptom, mood, sleep, and diet tracking and more.

Premom

This ovulation tracker measures one's luteinizing hormone (LH) surge to best predict ovulation.

Male Infertility

Podcasts

Fertility Docs Uncensored: Episode 6, "It's Not Just a Women's Problem—Exploring Male Infertility," and Episode 37, "Don't Forget about the Guys—All about Male Infertility"

In this podcast, fertility doctors Carrie Bedient, Abby Eblen, and Susan Hudson educate their audience by busting the common myths about infertility. Episode 6 covers male infertility in particular. In Episode 37, the hosts interview Dr. Chris Schrepferman, a Louisville urologist with specialized training in male infertility.

As a Woman: "Male Infertility, with Dr. Tolu Bakare," September 20, 2020

Dr. Natalie Crawford hosts this podcast about "fertility, hormones, and beyond." In the above episode, she interviews Dr. Tolu Bakare, a male infertility specialist, who tells the story of why she pursued medicine as well as lifestyle and medical facts regarding male infertility.

YouTube

Urology–Infertility (https://youtu.be/F4hkhmjzGD0)

Dr. Alexander Pastuzsak provides the need-to-know concepts of male infertility and what all goes into the approach to the infertile male in this two-and-a-half-minute video.

Reproductive Immunology

Podcasts

Fab Fertility: "A Reproductive Immunology Success Story w/ Author Hollie Overton," March 10, 2021

Author Hollie Overton shares her IVF success story.

Blogs

Pregmune (https://pregmune.com/blog/fertility-through-reproductive -immunology/)

Pregmune, a reproductive health technology company established by Dr. Andrea Vidali, has a blog, Finding Fertility Answers through Reproductive Immunology, that discusses fertility assessment. Check out their frequently asked questions for more information on reproductive immunology.

Sexual Dysfunction

Podcasts

Fertility Docs Uncensored: Episode 72, "'I'm Not in the Mood'—Low Libido in the Childbearing Years"

A thoughtful discussion about waning sexual desire as well as the treatments available.

You Are Not Broken: Season 1, Episodes 7 and 8

Host K. J. Casperson, MD, a female sexual function specialist, discusses low libido and available treatments. In these two episodes, she breaks down the pamphlet she hands out to patients at her practice regarding sexual dysfunction. She gives you all the information about desire (spontaneous and responsive), arousal, orgasmic dysfunction, and sexual pain concerns as well as treatment modalities.

Ask Dr. Drew: Episode 88, "What Causes Sexual Dysfunction?"

Board-certified urologist and male and female sexual dysfunction specialist Dr. Ashley Tapscott discuss the ins and outs of sexual dysfunction with host Dr. Drew Pinsky.

Websites

Up to Date (www.uptodate.com)

This website provides comprehensive information regarding the epidemiology, etiology, workup, diagnosis, and treatment of male sexual dysfunction.

YouTube

What Is Male Sexual Dysfunction? (https://youtu.be/h6PQaWySHrY)

Brought to you by Northwestern Medicine, this YouTube video featuring Dr. Nelson E. Bennett Jr., MD, urologist at Northwestern Memorial Hospital, discusses male sexual dysfunction, symptoms, and treatment options.

Understanding Female Sexual Dysfunction (https://youtu.be/Z6mC16Q0ZL8)

In this video from the American Sexual Health Association, clinical psychologist Sheryl Kingsberg, division chief of OB-GYN Behavioral Medicine at the University Hospitals Cleveland Medical Center, discusses the different types of female sexual dysfunction and how they impact our health and relationships.

Apps

Lover

> Developed in collaboration with sexual medicine clinical psychologist Dr. Britney Blair, this personalized, science-based app addresses various sexual concerns, providing assistance with erectile dysfunction and other sexual dysfunction.

Amenorrhea

Podcasts

As a Woman: "Amenorrhea Episode," February 23, 2020

> This episode features a discussion of the causes of both primary and secondary amenorrhea and a more thorough understanding of your menstrual cycle.

Medbullets Podcast: Season 1, Episode 106, and Season 1, Episode 236

> For the scientifically minded, this podcast offers a more in-depth medical explanation of both primary and secondary amenorrhea.

Abnormal Vaginal Bleeding

Podcasts

MediTalk: "Let's Talk Heavy Menstrual Bleeding (Menorrhagia) with Specialist Gynecologist Dr. Acton," July 9, 2020

> This podcast episode provides an explanation for heavy menstrual cycles and what may cause them, as well as the varying treatment options out there for women who suffer from irregular heavy bleeding.

CREOGs over Coffee: Episode 47, "Abnormal Uterine Bleeding"

> The hosts discuss the etiologies of abnormal uterine bleeding, including the popular mnemonic PALM-COEIN:

> P = polyp
> A = adenomyosis (endometrial-like tissue grows into wall of uterus)
> L = leiomyoma (fibroid)
> M = malignancy
> C = coagulopathy (abnormal blood clotting)
> O = ovulatory dysfunction (irregular periods)
> E = endometrial (problem in lining of uterus)
> I = iatrogenic (caused by treatment such as chemotherapy)
> N = not classified (other causes)

Endometriosis

Social Media

Instagram: @theendometriosisfoundation

An Instagram page dedicated to providing information and advocating for individuals with endometriosis. The foundation's envisions a future where endometriosis is better recognized and understood. Through this Instagram page, the foundation provides a link to their other resources, including a symptom diary, Facebook page and support group, YouTube channel, and Twitter account. Also included are videos of individuals sharing their personal experience with endometriosis, creating a great community feel to ensure women with this diagnosis do not feel alone.

MyEndometriosisTeam

MyEndometriosisTeam is a social networking app for women with endometriosis. In the app they can share experiences, ask questions, and connect with one another.

Facebook: Endo Warriors Group

This is a public support group for women to share their experiences with endometriosis, ask questions, and learn about upcoming events.

Podcasts

Fertility Docs Uncensored: Episode 10, "'The Jelly Belongs inside the Donut'—All about Endometriosis"

This episode is about all things endometriosis, including new developments in research and treatment of this complex condition.

YouTube

Endometriosis: Pathology, Symptoms, Risk Factors, Diagnosis and Treatment (https://youtu.be/GfrgbtXRCHw)

This video from Alila Medical Media provides a simple overview of endometriosis and what this diagnosis entails.

Polycystic Ovaries

Social Media

MyPCOSteam

Connect with thousands of members of this social media support group, primarily for individuals with PCOS.

Twitter: @PCOSAA

> For the Twitter users out there, this is the PCOS Awareness Association's account, which advocates for the PCOS community and provides information, resources, and support.

Podcasts

Fertility Docs Uncensored: Episode 28, "The Mysteries of PCOS—About Polycystic Ovary Syndrome"

> This episode explores PCOS, from diagnosis to treatment.

The Fertile Life with Dr. Shahin Ghadir: "What Is PCOS?" October 21, 2021

> In this episode, Dr. Shahin Ghadir provides a great overview of what constitutes the diagnosis of PCOS, including clinical signs and symptoms, what is seen on lab work, and how PCOS affects fertility.

The OBGYN Podcast: Episode 22, "PCOS"

> Join host Joseph Chappelle, MD, to learn about the history of polycystic ovarian syndrome, learn about the underlying physiology, and how it is diagnosed.

Uterine Fibroids

Podcasts

Fertility Docs Uncensored: Episode 18: "'Size Matters'—All about Fibroids"

> This episode thoroughly explains uterine fibroids, examining their diagnosis and treatment as well.

Natural MD Radio: Episode 150, "Uterine Fibroids: What Every Woman Needs to Know"

> Here the hosts discuss all things fibroids, including epidemiology, etiology, prevention, treatments, and more.

Videos

Fibroid Tumors: A Patient Education Video (www.reproductivefacts.org/resources/ educational-videos/videos/full-length-videos/videos/fibroid-tumors/)

> Recently diagnosed with a fibroid or just looking to understand common gynecologic topics? This educational video from the American Society of Reproductive Medicine goes the extra mile to discuss fibroids, their signs and symptoms, and how this diagnosis affects fertility.

Miscarriages

Podcasts

Fertility Docs Uncensored: Episode 34, "Hope after Heartbreak—Diagnosing and Treating Recurrent Pregnancy Loss"

A discussion of recurrent pregnancy loss, its causes, and available treatments.

Ectopic Pregnancy

Podcasts

As a Woman: Ectopic Pregnancy Episode, January 26, 2020

Host Natalie Crawford, MD, discusses the risk factors, diagnosis, and treatment options for an ectopic pregnancy.

Fertility Docs Uncensored: Episode 98, "Life after Ectopic Pregnancy"

Dr. Carrie Bedient, Dr. Abby Eblen, and Dr. Susan Hudson discuss what can cause an ectopic pregnancy, how doctors treat it, and what it means for future pregnancy attempts.

Assisted Reproductive Technology

Podcasts

Fertility Docs Uncensored: Episode 26: "The ABCs of IVF—Speaking the Language of Fertility"

This episode helps explain and familiarize some of the terms and lingo that one might hear during their IVF cycle.

YouTube

How In Vitro Fertilization (IVF) Works (https://youtu.be/P27waC05Hdk)

With the use of incredible visuals, Nassim Assefi and Brian A. Levine detail the science behind making a "baby in a lab."

What Is IVF? A Fertility Doctor Explains In Vitro Fertilization (https://youtu.be/hYtr6UfRFCk)

In this video, Dr. Natalie Crawford breaks down IVF so that you can be better prepared and better understand this process.

IVF ICSI Procedure: Important Things You Need to Know (https://youtu.be/lvLwU9G1Oug)

InfertilityTV produced this video, which demonstrates the intracytoplasmic sperm injection (ICSI) process and explains how it differs from standard insemination.

Preimplantation Genetic Testing (https://mountsinaifertility.com/fertility -treatments/pre-implantation-genetic-testing-monogenic-disease/)

A detailed explanation of the what, when, and how of PGT-A, along with an embedded YouTube video of the process, from Mount Sinai Infertility.

Social Egg Freezing

Podcasts

Fertility Docs Uncensored: Episode 89, "What's Egg Freezing Like? One Fertility Doctor's Experience"

This particular episode explores Dr. Meghan Smith's experience with freezing her own eggs.

Cancer and Fertility Preservation

Podcasts

Fertility Docs Uncensored: Episode 87, "Preserving the Dream of Motherhood—Fertility Treatment and Breast Cancer"

A thoughtful discussion of the options available for newly diagnosed breast cancer patients, as well as patients who have previously had breast cancer and are interested in having a baby.

Fertility Docs Uncensored: Episode 23: "'Highs and Lows'—Fertility Treatment for Cancer Patients"

Oncofertility (fertility preservation for patients with cancer) is discussed in this episode, which covers future options for individuals whose fertility may be affected by cancer and its subsequent treatment modalities.

The OB/GYN Podcast: Episode 32, "Oncofertility and Fertility Preservation"

Dr. Jillian Kurtz walks through the methods and rationale behind fertility preservation for patients with cancer or undergoing transgender procedures in this episode.

LGBTQ Couples and Fertility

Podcasts

Fertility Docs Uncensored: Episode 11, "Becoming Two Moms—LGBTQ Family Building"; Episode 71, "Helping Two Moms Conceive—Family-Building for

Same-Sex Couples"; and Episode 74, "Two Dads and a Baby—Family-Building for Same-Sex Male Couples"

The journey of family building as a lesbian couple is explored in Episode 11. Episode 71 offers an informative examination of the possibilities for same-sex female couples regarding family-building, donor sperm intrauterine insemination, and reciprocal IVF. In Episode 74, the hosts discuss the options for same-sex male couples for family-building, including but not limited to adoption, egg donation and gestational surrogacy, sperm collection, and embryo transfer.

The OB/GYN Podcast: Episode 32, "Oncofertility and Fertility Preservation"

Dr. Jillian Kurtz walks through the methods and rationale behind fertility preservation for patients with cancer or undergoing transgender procedures in this episode.

Military Fertility Services

Podcasts

Fertility Docs Uncensored: Episode 14, "Fighting to Become a Mother—Fertility Care for Military Professionals"

Testimony from a patient regarding her personal experience as a woman in the military and her own journey with fertility treatment is featured in this episode.

Managing Stress

Podcasts

Infertility Feelings: Season 1, Episode 41, "Stress, Anxiety, and Infertility"

Dr. Andrea Ganahl breaks down how we know if we are dealing with stress or anxiety when struggling to conceive. This episode is for anyone who has felt stressed or anxious during their experience with infertility.

YouTube

How to Tap with Jessica Ortner: Emotional Freedom Technique Informational Video (https://youtu.be/pAclBdj20ZU)

This informational video discusses the functional medicine technique of tapping.

Apps

Noom

> This smartphone app is designed to instill healthier habits to manage stress and anxiety.

Calm

> On-the-go app with meditations, lessons, and soothing sounds to help one conquer stress, anxiety, sleeping difficulties, depression, and the various challenges of day-to-day life.

Financing the Infertility Journey

Podcasts

Fertility Docs Uncensored: Episode 15, "Finances and Fertility—Covering the Cost of Fertility Treatment"

> The hosts have a thorough conversation about the costs for fertility treatment, including diagnostic and treatment coverage, as well as copay and deductible cost.

Donor Insemination

Podcasts

Fertility Docs Uncensored: Episode 42, "'1 in 100 Guys'—All about Anonymous Sperm Donation"

> This episode details the process of anonymous sperm donation, highlighting the requirements a sperm donor must fulfill to be considered for this process.

Pregnancy

Podcasts

All about Pregnancy and Birth

> This podcast describes itself as your place for supportive, evidence-based information from Dr. Nicole Calloway Rankins, an OB-GYN who's been in practice for nearly 15 years and has helped bring more than 1,000 babies into this world.

YouTube

Getting Pregnant: Everything You Need to Know (Tips from a Fertility Doctor) (https://youtu.be/coJACcnOSRQ)

This quick, eight-minute video led by a fertility doc at Shady Grove Infertility discusses the do's and don'ts, tips and tricks, and myths of getting pregnant.

Apps
BabyCenter

> Track all stages of pregnancy weekly, including symptoms, fetus size, informative tips, and support from others expecting at the same time through this smartphone app.

Ovia

> App committed to providing support for families and expectant mothers, offering information about pregnancy milestones, symptoms, nutrition, doctor appointments, and mood.

The Bump Pregnancy Tracker

> Rated the best for new moms, this pregnancy tracker app provides a one-stop shop for all things pregnancy, including expected symptoms, a tailored timeline, size comparisons, and fetal development information. This app also has the unique feature of a weekly checklist of tasks to complete leading up to baby's arrival.

Index

ginger: as remedy for morning sickness, 182

gonadotropin-releasing hormone (GnRH), 65, 66, 67

gonorrhea: as risk factor for ectopic pregnancy, 109

hair growth (in women): as symptom of PCOS, 86, 89

Hashimoto's thyroiditis, 27, 48

Health Care Fairness for Military Act, 156

health care insurance: and coverage for infertility diagnosis and treatment, 165–66, 167

helper T1 and T2 assay, 50

hemochromatosis, 65

herbal supplements, 16

high blood pressure: treatment of, during pregnancy, 17

high-intensity focused ultrasound (HIFU) ablation: of uterine fibroids, 75

hirsutism. *See* hair growth (in women)

human chorionic gonadotropin (HCG): as hormone measured in pregnancy tests, 111, 180

human menopausal gonadotropin (HMG), 31

human trafficking: and gestational carrying, 176

hydrocele, 37, 38

hyperemesis gravidarum, 182

hyperprolactinemia, 65

hyperthyroidism, 17

hypogonadism, 37

hypogonadotropic hypogonadism, 65–66; idiopathic, 67

hypospadias, 41–42

hypothalamic-pituitary-ovarian axis, 65, 66

hypothyroidism, 17

hysterectomy: as treatment for abnormal vaginal bleeding, 74; as treatment for adenomyosis, 80

hysterosalpingogram (HSG), 117

hysteroscopic myomectomy, 98, 152

hysteroscopy, 31, 71, 98, 105

idiopathic hypogonadotropic hypogonadism (IHH), 67

immune system: and pregnancy, 48–52

immunologic infertility, 52, 187; and dietary changes, 50; tests for, 49–50; treatment of, 50, 52

impotence, 42. *See also* infertility, male; sexual dysfunction

incompetent cervix: as risk factor for miscarriage, 104

infection: as risk factor for miscarriage, 104

infertility, female, 33; age as factor in, 27, 28; anatomical causes of, 26–27; blood tests relating to, 29; cancer therapy drugs as risk for, 140–41; causes of, 25–28, 186–87; costs of treatment for, 164–69; and endometriosis, 80; evaluation for, 28–29; and immune system, 48–50; medical conditions affecting, 27–28; personal experiences relating to, 1–11, 22, 32–33, 46–47, 50–52, 63, 70–71, 77–78, 81–83, 85, 90–91, 93, 98–99, 101, 106–7, 108–9, 113–15,

Kaplan, Helen Singer, 55
Kinsey Institute, 55
Klinefelter syndrome, 37, 41
Kruger criteria, 36

laparascopic surgery: as treatment for
    endometriosis, 77
laparoscopy, 29; and diagnosis of
    endometriosis, 80
LEEP (loop electrosurgical excision
    procedure), 26
leiomyoma. *See* uterine fibroids
Lending Club Patient Solutions, 168
letrozole (Femara), 31, 32, 67; as
    treatment for PCOS, 88, 91
Levitra, 57
LGBTQ couples: fertility treatment
    options for, 145–51, 188; personal
    experiences relating to, 149–50
lifestyle choices (diet and exercise):
    changes in, as treatment for PCOS,
    88, 90; and a healthy pregnancy, 15,
    21, 43, 106, 153, 154, 180–82
Livestrong Fertility Program, 19
loop electrosurgical excision procedure
    (LEEP), 26
lupus: impact of, on fertility, 27, 48; and
    pregnancy, 17
luteinizing hormone (LH), 14, 29, 65, 66,
    89, 129, 130; injections of, 68, 130
Lybrido/Lybridos, 58

macroadenoma, 69
magnesium, 180
magnetic resonance imaging (MRI): and
    diagnosis of uterine fibroids, 97

male hormones, elevated: as cause of
    amenorrhea, 65
marijuana: impact of, on fertility, 27, 37,
    40
Masters, William H., 55
maternal age, advanced, 25
medications: for abnormal vaginal
    bleeding, 73–74; for amenorrhea,
    67–68; for endometriosis, 81; for
    erectile dysfunction, 57; as factor in
    infertility, 37, 39–40; for PCOS,
    88–90; safety of, during pregnancy,
    17; for sexual dysfunction, 58; for
    uterine fibroids, 97
menopause: and amenorrhea, 64;
    premature, 64
menorrhagia (heavy periods), 71. *See also*
    vaginal bleeding, abnormal
menstruation, 65–67; personal experi-
    ences relating to, 63, 68–69;
    retrograde, 79. *See also* amenorrhea;
    vaginal bleeding, abnormal
mental health: and pregnancy, 19. *See also*
    stress
metformin (as treatment for PCOS), 89
methotrexate: as treatment for ectopic
    pregnancy, 112
metrorrhagia (bleeding between periods),
    71. *See also* vaginal bleeding,
    abnormal
military infertility services, 153, 154–55,
    158, 188; financial support offered
    by, 155–57; personal experiences
    relating to, 152, 157–58; treatment
    facilities, 154–55; treatment options
    available through, 155–57

pregnancy associated with, 86; diagnosis of, 86–87; diet and exercise as treatment for, 88, 90; and male hormones, 87; personal experiences relating to, 85, 90–91; prevalence of, 86; symptoms of, 86; tests for, 86–87; treatments for, 88–90

steviosides, 181

stress: coping with, 161; evaluation of, 160; as factor for active duty military personnel, 154; infertility as source of, 159–61; personal experiences relating to, 159, 161–62; treatment for, 160–61

Strickland, Marilyn, 157

submucosal fibroids, 94, 95, 98

subserosal fibroids, 95, 98

sugars: to be avoided during pregnancy, 180–81

surrogacy. *See* gestational carriers

Tay-Sachs disease, 29

teratozoospermia, 37, 38

testicles, undescended, 37, 41

testicular sperm extraction (TESE), 42–43

testicular torsion, 37, 38

testosterone therapy, 39

thrombophilia. *See* blood clots

thyroid disorders: and amenorrhea, 65; and pregnancy, 17; as risk factor for miscarriage, 103; tests relating to, 29, 72

thyroiditis, 27

thyroid stimulating hormone (TSH), 17, 29

tibolone, 58

toxins. *See* environmental toxins

tranexamic acid: as treatment for abnormal vaginal bleeding, 73

transgender men: fertility preservation for, 145–48; surrogacy and adoption as options for, 148

transgender patients: fertility preservation for, 145–51; multidisciplinary approach recommended for, 146; personal experiences relating to, 145–46, 149–50; social stigma experienced by, 148

transgender women: fertility preservation for, 147–48

transman, 147. *See also* transgender men

transsexual, 147

transwoman, 147. *See also* transgender women

TRICARE benefits: for military infertility services, 153, 156–57

triploidy, 104

tubal surgery: as risk factor for ectopic pregnancy, 110

ulcerative colitis: impact of, on fertility, 27

ultrasound: and diagnosis of uterine fibroids, 96–97

undescended testes, 37, 41

unicornuate uterus, 33

urologists: and male infertility, 36

uterine artery embolization (UAE), 98

uterine fibroids (leiomyoma), 27, 30, 31, 93–94, 99–100; and abnormal vaginal bleeding, 70–71, 72, 73, 74, 75–76; diagnosis of, 96–97; location of, 94–95; medications for, 97; personal experiences relating to, 93, 98–99; and pregnancy complications, 94–95; race as factor in, 94; as risk factor for miscarriage, 104; surgery for removal of, 74; symptoms of, 96; treatments for, 97–98, 152

About the Authors

Joseph S. Sanfilippo, MD, MBA

Joseph S. Sanfilippo, MD, MBA, is a tenured professor of obstetrics, gynecology, and reproductive sciences and the vice chair of Reproductive Sciences at the University of Pittsburgh School of Medicine, Magee-Womens Hospital. There, he is the academic director of the Division of Reproductive Endocrinology and Infertility and has directed Fellowship training programs in reproductive endocrine infertility for more than two decades. A Distinguished Alumnus of the Rosalind Franklin University of Medicine and Science at Chicago Medical School, he has been named a "Top Doctor" for over 20 consecutive years and is the recipient of a Lifetime Achievement in Gynecology Award. He has also published numerous textbooks in obstetrics and gynecology. Dr. Sanfilippo is a previous executive director of the North American Society for Pediatric and Adolescent Gynecology, an emeritus editor-in-chief of the *Journal of Pediatric and Adolescent Gynecology*, and a past president of the American Society for Reproductive Medicine and the Society for Reproductive Surgeons. His clinical interests include pediatric and adolescent gynecology, minimally invasive surgery, and reproductive endocrinology and infertility.

Aarti Kumar, MD

Aarti Kumar, MD, graduated from the University of Pittsburgh School of Medicine in 2021. There, she served four years as the vice president of the student body. Dr. Kumar was a recipient of the Chancellor's Scholarship and earned her BA in sociology from the University of Pittsburgh, where she graduated from the Honors College and was inducted into the Phi Beta Kappa Society in 2017. A member of the American College of Obstetricians and Gynecologists and the Society of Gynecologic Oncology, she has published articles in the *Journal of Neurocritical Care* and the *Annals of Infertility and Reproductive Endocrinology*. Presently, Dr. Kumar is an OB-GYN resident at NYU Langone Health, where she is a bilingual provider.